ERIC ROBESPIERRE

I0101930

Cracking
the
Walnut

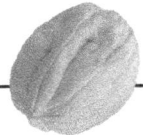

How Being a Little Nuts

Helped Me to Beat Prostate Cancer

To the survivors

I would like to thank my loving family and caring friends, as well as, the nurses and my doctors for their dedicated professionalism, unwavering support and for putting up with my craziness. Special thanks go to Sarah Coots, my brilliant editor, and to the equally gifted Victoria Jamieson, who designed the cover.

It is my hope that my story will provide readers with similar support, as well as permission to act "a little nuts" if that's what it takes to get through this ordeal.

Library of Congress Control Number: 2010916824
ISBN 9780615416366

Published by Eric Robespierre
www.ericrobespierre.com

ROUND 1

DON'T let anyone tell you digging up a grave is easy. So—what in the world am I doing at a gravesite, in the pitch of night, on my hands and knees, feverishly clawing at the dirt, buckets of rain pouring down, soaking me to the bone? I want to murder my father, kill him for passing down deadly genetic material to his only son. He gave me life, but I'm pissed to the brim he had the hereditary right to take it back.

I'm only kidding. Revenge may be best served up cold, but I'm not crazy enough to actually dig up my dear old dead dad—that's morbidly sick, or a good opening for a Romero scare job. More to the point, I love my father. I miss him terribly. Let me prove it: Say God, in all his infinite glory, magically appears before me and says, "Eric Robespierre—I like you, always have, always will—so here's the deal, kid. How' bout a new Papaw, only this one'll be good to the walnut?"

You know what I would reply once I regained consciousness? "How come you look like Charlton Heston, but sound like Elvis?" Just kidding. I'd say, "Thanks—but no thanks." Respectfully, of course—you don't mouth off against the Big Guy. I'd also take the opportunity to give Him a shout-out for keeping my Stuyvesant Town apartment rent stabilized.

I talk this way now, still glib, still unsure what the urologist will discover, but should my rising PSA (prostate specific antigen) numbers climb to the level of the unthinkable, well then—in today's argot—I'd be royally fucked, maybe actually lose it enough to head out to Cemetery Central and do a Romero on Daddy Dearest. Who knows, I might not even return.

Let's face it: when the horse has left the barn, what choice do you have but to bend over and kiss your sorry ass goodbye? Doing a kiss-off in a cemetery has a kick-ass ring to it; makes things so much more convenient and cheaper for those you left behind, don't you think?

It's time to open my eyes, get out of bed and put an end to ghoulish thoughts, because the longer I lay here in my Brothers *Grim* twilight, the more I drive myself nuttier, and nuttier and nuttier.

My perversity reminds me of those neurotic times when I have a tiny, but bothersome splinter in my finger—I know when I touch it, no matter how gently, it will hurt, yet instead of taking Rational Road and simply refraining from fingering it until I can do some sterile self-surgery, I take Nut Case Walk and cannot suppress the desire to press down on the soft, tender flesh, again and again and again, each time incrementally increasing the pain that inexorably radiates up the inflamed area and into my hand. Fortunately, I don't get too many splinters.

Time to seek out some music—the best thing to calm my neurotic *breast* (owning up to onanism not withstanding). I learned this first as a ten-year-old with Doo Wop: "Deserie," by the Charts; "Over The Mountain," by Johnny and Joe. Then at thirteen, it was rock and roll: Big Haley, The Fat Man, Little Richard, Bo Diddley, and the King. Then jazz in college: Blakey, Ramsey, J.J. Johnson, and Miles—Miles of Miles; classical in grad school: Beethoven, Mahler, Mozart; and finally, in my thirties, opera: Verdi, Puccini, Wagner—a world of thrilling harmonies and vocal gymnastics.

I often play the same piece at the same time of the day for a week, month, five months. Right now, mornings belong to the pianist Dinu Lipatti playing a selection of Bach, Mozart, Scarlatti, and Schubert—mood-altering harmonies guaranteed to release my lovely pal Dopamine and bathe me in a mind-soaking chemical bliss.

But today it doesn't seem to be working.

Wait. I have another kind of a soak that might do it: a long, hot, tub bath, another neurological happy pill that usually calms my crazies. I get in and feel my pores open in a quasi-religious welcome. The waters are warm and soothing, but unfortunately, my troubled mind is doomsday-racing with anxiety. I can't soak still.

I've left the door open so I can hear the music. Perhaps, if I close my eyes and let the music and the water wash over me, the combination will calm me. It's the rhythmically intoxicating "Partita for Keyboard No. 1 in B-flat major," by Bach; for a moment my brain is hijacked. Angst is flushed down the drain, and I'm floating in a rhapsody of tranquility—until workmen arrive below my window, and a series of staccato thumps and whumps that travel upwards with the explosiveness of a 747 taking off shatter my serenity.

In desperation, I try submerging my head (holding my nose, of course), pretending I'm diving for pearls or maybe looking to break the Guinness World Records for Nostril-Holding in a Five-Foot, Post-War, Porcelain-Peeling Tub, covered head to foot in a protective wet suit. Or perhaps daring to do the stunt *sans* suit, covered only by a thick, greasy jell impervious to New York City bacteria. Envisioning such a sports moment, however risky it would be, normally distracts me in troubled waters.

But not today.

I think about going for another kind of record—say consecutive dunks without breathing, maybe five, ten, in a skintight Speedo. It's a maneuver I've never attempted, but a derring-do worth the risk.

Not today.

I know what's bothering me. Lying in the tub, peering over my naked body half-submerged in the brackish (courtesy of fifty-year-old pipes) water, I can't help but stare at Mr. Floppy, AKA Mr. Stiffy (in better times). He's obviously not the problem, but offensive nevertheless because he symbolizes the crisis. Oh, and don't tell me Mr. Floppy doesn't know the score, bobbing limply in the murky water, laying low, trying to avoid attention, hoping to hell I won't shoot the messenger because I don't like the message.

I raise myself up to a standing position in the tub—carefully, so as not to slip and break my neck. Fear may be the mind-killer, but it'll also distract your ass and make you fall and break it. I turn on the shower, stick my face directly into the showerhead, and feel the sting as my skin yells, *Too fucking hot!* My cheeks burn, my nose closes up, and I hold my breath for as long as I can—maybe another Guinness Record?

Nope, not today.

Well—at least the pain is somewhat distracting. Now for a good soap-it-up with stuff I got in bulk from Costco that smells a little too *tutti frutti*, flaring my nostrils as it taunts the masculinity of my nose. Unlike Mr. Floppy, my sniffer is unaware of any looming doom, and is still hard as a rock. (This *tutti frutti* soap is a product I normally wouldn't purchase, but like the other Jewish dilemma—pork on sale—was too good to pass up.)

I then give myself a cooling coconut shampoo out of a bottle that must weigh fifty pounds (another Costco saver), but thank God it doesn't smell like ladies (you just have to *look* at a hairy coconut to know it's ballsy), rub-a-dub-dubbing soap and shampoo until the foamy whiteness completely covers the brown waters and gives me the illusion that I'm not bathing in sewage. I follow up with a little three-sixty rinse-a-dinse under the showerhead.

I slowly get myself out of the tub without doing a header onto the tiles (I'm still in my *fear-is-the-mind-killer*/ass-breaker mode). However, before my cautious exit, I make damn sure I gently lather Mr. Floppy with reverential care. *I know it's not your fault, and whatever happens*, I say to him silently, *just remember we'll get through it together.* I hope for a salute in response.

Not today.

I dry myself off and then dart naked into the living room to make the music a tad lower. I don't want jealous market-rate neighbors complaining, giving management another reason to rid them of the dreaded rent-stabilized tenant. I unconsciously cover my privates as I glance furtively out my window and across the courtyard at the apartments facing me, looking for any movement that might indicate a neighbor, a peeper, anyone looking to post voyeuristic photos of me on YouTube. I don't spot anything perverted, and just as quickly scamper back to the bathroom. Empowered by my daring, and suddenly full of stones, I momentarily care nothing about having the shakes, and begin to shave my smiley face.

I stare in the mirror. "I told you I could do it, pally."

The recognizable face in the mirror grins back: thin, scarred lips parted ever so slightly; jaw line square and chiseled granite hard; grey fedora pulled neatly down over the disfigured half-moon eyebrows, leaving a straight shadow across a nose that's been shaped by one too many knuckle sandwiches. Good old Philip Marlowe, my get-tough persona when times get tough.

"Come on, finish up, pally; let's dangle."

No scrapes, no cuts, no nicking the tips of the nose. A real bleeding bitch when that happens. Shaving malpractice requires a good smear of Vaseline and an ugly wad of tissue paper—the Vaseline being the key, or else look out, because no matter how gently you pull off the paper, there will be blood.

I dress myself without mismatching socks, sneakers, or mixing plaids with stripes, but there's just so much bravado you can get from forty seconds of running naked into your living room, and when the adrenaline rush is gone, the anguish that began two short days ago again descends, in the familiar form of a smothering black cloud that threatens to become my second skin. What better time than now to tell you how this all started?

Traditional slow fade should take us through the cloud. Yes—here we are, only two short days ago: Monday, October 8, 10:30 a.m.

"Déjà *blue* all over again, boys and girls."

I'm busy as a little bee working on a new book about my "romantic" journey into the world of online dating—a trip that alternates between comedy and tragedy—when the phone rings and brings me out of the writer's world of make believe and into the unpleasant unmanageability of everyday reality. The caller ID identifies my doctor, and I instantaneously compute that he's on the line with the results of my annual checkup. *Hold it uno momento, Masked Man—that doesn't compute!* I always have to call *him*; Dr. Lombardo never calls *me*. I grab my half-full coffee cup and take a comforting swallow.

"Eric—this is Dr. Lombardo . . ."

No nurse to say, *Hold on, it's Dr. Lombardo*, a nice touch that could add precious milliseconds, allow my fragile brain to hunker down before synapses jump the rails and disconnect in a blaze of exploding white light.

"Shit!"

He tells me my cholesterol is okay, as are my liver functions, but my PSA levels are up from last year to three-point-nine-one, so he wants me to see the urologist.

"Shit, shit, and double-shit!"

Dr. Lombardo tempers the news by reassuring me that my good antigens are good (whatever that means) and I shouldn't worry. Obviously, he hasn't a clue as to whom he's talking, otherwise, he would have had someone from the Suicide Prevention Hotline listening in; better still, two burly men in white by my side, ready to shoot me full of Thorazine, not that that would have been enough to put me out of my misery. Remember how Roy Scheider kills the shark in *Jaws*? Probably nothing less than a barrel of exploding dynamite down my throat would do the trick. Dr. Lombardo babbles on, but I'm not hearing a thing.

"Fear is the mind-killer", and I'm waiting for the rest of my body to catch up to my dead brain, but amazingly I'm not experiencing any of the usual suspects: sweats, heart palpitations, throat closings, hands trembling, out-of-body wanderings (usually watching myself being buried alive).

I'm just repeating *Shit, Shit, Shit* over and over in my head. Maybe my mind hasn't really been atomized, but simply gone into Shit Lockdown. Somehow I gain control of my vocal cords and speak. I surprise myself; my voice is clear and forceful.

"I've never been to the urologist."

I would like Dr. Lombardo—a very cool guy who loves to read, like me—to reply, "Well, Eric, in that case—forgetaboutit." Instead, it's a scene right out of the *Body Snatchers*. Oh, it may be my doc's voice, but I know it's not him.

"What insurance do you have?"

An alien from Planet HMO! Okay, Eric, deal with it.

"Medicare and AARP."

Bravo! Instantaneously I'm clicked over to his receptionist (also body snatched) and must repeat the info before she looks through her list and gives me the urologist who takes my insurance.

I write down the doctor's name and phone number and repeat it back.

Although she's doing a really good imitation and would have the ordinary person fooled, I've seen enough abduction movies to know what planet she makes home.

I hang up. I stare at the pad. The fucking phone call is real—it's time to meet the Ferryman.

"Shit, shit, double-shit!"

I have to break this loop.

"Stop, stop, double-stop!"

I've tricked my brain. Can't run two sound loops at the same time.

Coffee—I need coffee. My cup's empty. *Any more left? Let me think.* Well, that's a useless exercise at this point, so I go into the kitchen. The coffee pot is dry as a bone. I have to make more, however, this time I'll double up and make it really strong. I stare at the open bottle of Crane Lake Merlot. What I really want—need—is a glass of wine, a big glass of red wine. 10:45 a.m.! Ahh, what the hell—a dead man's last request. *Go for it!* one part of me says. And then, *Are you nuts?*

I stare at the square-jawed reflection in the microwave window.

"Don't be a sucker, pally. You don't need to gargle now."

I could argue that somewhere in the world it's a reasonable time to drink—the Philippines for one—but Marlowe isn't buying it, okay?

As I make my brew, I look at the bright side: I'm not doing a St. Vitus dance in the middle of my kitchen, but at least I remembered to put in the water before turning on Mr. Coffee. Fear is not only the mind-killer and ass-breaker, but also the leading cause of Mr. Coffee deaths. I begin to take my vitamins, which includes Saw Palmetto, a supplement promoted as supporting prostate health. I think about taking twice the dosage, but then stop. Why not? Is it too late? Has the horse really left the barn? Will taking the extra pill be positive admission something may be wrong, ergo if I don't, I can fool my body into thinking everything is okay? But . . . taking the pill is a good thing, and taking two will be twice as good.

Sigmund Freud in the Vitamin Shoppe with an axe. Psycho migraine! Psycho migraine!

This inner dialogue is insane and only proves that either I have a split personality or that Hannity and Colmes have taken over my body. I stare at the Crane Lake. *Stop it!* I take my vitamins and double up on the Saw Palmetto, washing it down with a gulp of vanilla soymilk. See—I take care of my body, I can't have bad walnuts. I pour the coffee into a cup with a large M on it; it was my father's. Why shouldn't it be? This was once his apartment; it is still his furniture, paintings, utensils, cups. Did he drink coffee out of this same cup the day he got the news his PSA scores might mean death and destruction, as they eventually did for him?

Camus in the cranium with my father's coffee mug! Existential migraine! Existential migraine!

"Shit, shit, triple-shit!"

The drilling outside suddenly starts up again, and I jump. I look out the kitchen window: They're tearing up the walkway in preparation for a repaving job. I go into the living room just as the Lipatti CD concludes. Time for more music, and louder—drown out the mind-altering drilling. I fish out some opera: Mozart, *The Abduction from The Seraglio.* The lively overture fills me with hope and gives me the courage I need.

I nervously dial the urologist and in two rings get through to a receptionist. I explain as lucidly and succinctly as possible my situation, making sure to tell her that I'm a patient of Dr. Lombardo's. I expect a long wait, but no—it's a minute at the most before she says there's an opening this coming Wednesday at 3:00 p.m. Without giving it a second thought, I agree.

The dutiful, double checking receptionist wants to know what medical insurance I have. *Get with the program, Eric. Don't you know everyone in the health-care system's been abducted? Didn't you pay attention to Hillary?* I tell her to hold on; no reply. I go into the bedroom, search for my wallet, can't believe it's in the first place I look, nervously rummage through the compartments, can't believe the cards are all together in the exact place my fingers go—maybe this is a sign, maybe the shit won't hit the fan. I return to the living room and give HMO Abductee the information. She wants to know if I know where the doctor is located.

"No. I don't know it."

She tells me the address. I immediately recognize the building: My ex-wife's grandmother lives there until she died, sometime back in the late Seventies. Up until that moment, I had only fond memories of it, but now visualizing Grandma Helen's beautiful façade and ornamental lobby fills me with dread.

I stare at the phone and it dawns on me that the appointment's two days from today. Two days! Doesn't it usually take a week, maybe two, to see a specialist?

Two days! That's a damn nod and a wink! Do I make the call to the urologist if I know they will take me so quickly? Then again, the sooner the better I see someone—right? Right! Everybody says that. Right? Right! The longer you put it off, the more you drive yourself nuts.

Right?

Right! everybody says with a jackhammer in my forebrain.

Health dilemma migraine! Health dilemma migraine!

"Shit, shit, and quadruple-shit."

In—what?—less than half an hour, my life is turned upside down. *Hold it! Not yet, cowboy. This may be nothing.* Okay—so I'm not *totally* upside down, just at a forty-five-degree tilt, but believe me, that's enough to throw me off balance and no way to live your life in a straight-up world. I finish my coffee, sit down, and try to get caught up in the opera. It takes all my effort to sit motionless on the couch and listen. I close my eyes and try to visualize Mozart conducting the orchestra as I remember it in *Amadeus*. What's the name of the actor? He was in *Animal House*. Think—think! Tom Hulce! Kruger! Pinto! TOGA! I leap up from the couch and jump around the room.

"TOGA, TOGA, TOGA!"

The overture ends, the opera begins, and I stand motionless in the middle of the room. What's next? I know: I turn off Mozart, grab a Led Zeppelin CD from the shelf, put in CD 1 of *How The West Was Won,* and go immediately to the second cut—"Immigrant Song." The opening wail releases me. I join in on the next one. I replay the opening wails two, three, four times.

I switch off the CD player, collapse on the couch. I have to tell someone. Who? My two grown children, Nicholas and Gillian? I love them both deeply, wish they were here right now so I could hug them, get some support; then again, why worry them when it might be nothing? To call or not to call . . . Probably—but not just yet.

I think of calling my former writing partner, Helen, who now owns and operates a gym. She's a good friend, and one who knows all there is to know about health issues. Helen also knows how to set me straight when I get testy or a little nuts (no puns intended). She also has a knack for calming me when I get down and want to beat myself up with a meat cleaver. To call or not to call . . . Probably—but not just yet.

What about my former girlfriend? We're still friends, and she's definitely the most composed and serene person I know. In fact, she's the one who taught me to meditate. I know if I unburden myself to her she'll only fill me with positive energy. To call or not to call . . . Probably—but not just yet.

Then there's my childhood friend Werner, another positive thinker, steeped in Buddhism, and a person who will, no doubt, also have a calming effect when I unload my shit on him. In the last two years he has been my closest male friend and one with whom I've shared secrets, fears, misgivings, crass humor—a dialogue provoking more insightful breakthroughs than any ten shrinks or daily acid drops could possibly provide (okay, maybe not the acid drop). To call or not to call . . . Probably—but not just yet.

No—the person I am calling is my good friend Ira. Why Ira? Because two years ago Ira was diagnosed with bad walnuts, and after undergoing radiation and seed implants appears to be totally cured.

I dial up his number. We haven't talked in a while, and I feel guilty for that, and for the fact I'm calling him because I need him. But that's stupid—that's what friends are for. Right? Right! I call his office. Great!—he's in, and the receptionist puts me through. Right away he apologizes for not calling me, readily admits he's terrible at keeping in touch and tells me how he feels really guilty. I tell him I'm just as guilty for not checking up on him on a regular basis. If this were a girlie movie, they'd bring up the Beyoncé, but it isn't—instead Ira wants to set something up for next week, and we agree on Wednesday at 6:30 p.m. He insists I call him the day before to remind him and make sure we're still on.

"So—Ira—how are you?"

So innocuous this salutation appears when we expect an equally harmless response, only with Ira neither the question nor the answer is innocent, not after you learn he's got bad walnuts—then "How are you?" really means "How's the battle for your life going?" Over the last year or so, Ira's response has always been positive, and if I ever doubted his word, I saw for myself how well he was doing when we met for dinner outside the long, white, windowless building where moments before he'd undergone a radiation treatment. At a restaurant a few blocks away, he ate and drank with unbridled enthusiasm, and I couldn't detect the slightest side effects from either the treatment or the disease.

But that was then. Now is now. Now we tag on yet another hidden meaning to "How are you?" This time it's not just about him—it's about *me*, because I'm now saying to myself, *If he's not good, not really not cured—what hope do I have?*

Ira says, "Fine, everyone's fine;" my friend's words are crisp and clear. I let out a sigh of relief I hope he doesn't hear. He wants to know about me, especially about how the online dating scene is progressing. I want to brush off the questions and get right to my problem, but I force myself to hide the fear, (*Fear is the mind-killer,* I repeat to myself), and provide a lively and humorous description of my recent failures, as well as a synopsis of the book I'm currently writing. This takes extreme effort on my part, and I sense the hollowness in my voice. I hope Ira doesn't notice.

After my forced recital, I realize I'm not going to get the opening I need to allow me to segue smoothly into the real reason for my call, so I simply blurt it out: "I just had my annual checkup and my PSA scores went up and I've got to see an urologist."

There is no "Ah, shit" or any emotional outburst, Ira simply wants to know my numbers.

I quickly check my pad. Thank God I had the presence of mind to write them down, though, for the life of me, I don't remember doing so. Ira doesn't know the exact number that sent him off to the urologist, but he thinks it's around seven.

"Yours is lower. I wouldn't worry. It may be nothing. PSA numbers go up as we get older."

"There's my silver lining."

"Or it may be an infection—that can cause it to go up, too."

I'm encouraged by his remarks—encouraged? Hell, I'm ready to scream for joy. He asks if I have any symptoms and I quickly say no, without knowing what symptoms he means.

As if reading my mind, he continues, "You know—burning when you urinate, frequent urination and fever."

I immediately respond with a series of no's, hoping this will cut short what is now turning into a really disagreeable conversation. *"Fear is the mind-killer, fear is the mind-killer."* This is better than saying, *Shit, shit, double-shit.*

I name my urologist, hoping he's Ira's doc, but it's not going to happen:

"I've seen a lot of guys, but I don't remember this guy. You know my memory's shot; maybe Sharon would remember his name. But anyway, the guy I ended up with is Dr. Berman."

I'm thinking of asking for Berman's address, just in case he might be in the same office, but Ira's rushing to a meeting and has to jump.

"Don't worry, it's probably nothing. Just call me when you know something. See ya next week."

"Yep, I will call you."

Sure, Ira gave me information that encourages me to momentarily believe I might not have bad walnuts, but his reassurances aren't lasting, and certainly not powerful enough to jump-start my locked-down brain. Strange, though, that besides my numbness there are still no physical signs of anxiety. I know—I'll have a glass of wine.

At high noon (no pun intended), I pour out a handful of almonds, and cut open a Fuji apple and a nice big piece of Jarlsberg. The only thing missing is the French bread—and my PSA score being normal. Hey, plenty of execs have a cocktail or two at lunch. Well, okay—I've seen *Lost Weekend*; maybe this is the start of something I can't handle, but on the other hand, maybe a little buzz takes the edge off, and like the song says, helps me make it through the night.

The phone rings. It's my friend Ellyn. Ira must have called his wife, Sharon, and she must have called her sister. I've known Ellyn since the mid-Eighties, when we both worked at Grey Advertising. It was Ellyn who introduced me to Ira and Sharon. At first I resisted. I'm basically shy, reluctant to meet new people, but Ellyn's persuasiveness convinced me to meet her brother-in law, her saying there was no doubt in her mind Ira and I would get along great. A time came when Ira needed marketing and advertising work for his cake business, so we finally met. It took a while (Ira's just as shy and guarded), but eventually we became good friends. Then Ira sold his business, so we don't see each other as much as before, but when we do, we pick up the conversation as if we had just met the day before.

Whenever I mention how much I like Ira, Ellyn always says, "Well, I told you so." I always respond by saying, "You're right." In fact, Ellyn's always right. I think she's simply blessed with more common sense than most of us—except when it comes to bringing home and keeping the dogs she rescues, the numbers sometimes exceeding the space she has in her home and the time she has available to walk and care for each. Fortunately for Ellyn, her husband, Rob, is a saint, or at least has the patience of one when it comes to putting up with the mayhem these dogs constantly create.

Ellyn's also the one with her finger on everything medical. Not only does she work for a doctor, she also has a slew of doctor friends who provide her with referrals, so naturally when Ira's PSA went up, it was Ellyn who set him up with a new urologist, then an oncologist, both of whom she said were tops in their field. If this wasn't enough, Ellyn and Sharon do tons of research on bad walnuts, and stay on top of Ira's course of treatment.

Because of her expertise, and the fact she's also a trusted confidante, it's my intention to call Ellyn—right after I fortify myself with some *vino*—but she beats me to it.

The sound of her voice is reassuring, and her first words tell me I'm right in assuming Sharon via Ira alerted Ellyn to my condition.

"How are you feeling?"

For the first time since hearing the news I come clean.

"I'm scared." Just saying the words seems to free me.

Ellyn makes me repeat all the information I know, then provides an in-depth description of Ira's treatment. The upshot of it is, "Don't worry until you have something to worry about, but if it turns out to be prostate cancer, just remember, Ira's fine—you'll be fine." Ellyn makes me promise to call her as soon as I get the results of my next PSA.

"Prostrate cancer"—the death words blithely fall from her lips, and why not, she will never get it. But words are powerful things, and right now all you'll get from me is "bad walnuts"—a most welcomed euphemism—thanks to the prostate's nutty shape.

Flashback over! Now you have it! I'm feeling strangely calm after my total recall. Let me see, it's 8:00 a.m. Wow, that only took fifteen minutes? Well, there were omissions. Too much information can be boring to you and upsetting to me (I have a great habit of forgetting the really damaging-to-the-psyche stuff), but I think it's certainly enough to bring you and me up to speed.

I check myself out in the bedroom mirror: blue jeans, a little frayed at the cuffs; white long-sleeve dress shirt, open at the collar (couldn't close it if I wanted to) and hanging Brad Pitt-like over my jeans (to hide the little gut); on my feet, Thurlos and sneakers. I also decide to put on a sports jacket, and over that a lightweight, soft-as-butter, black leather coat my dad bought years ago at the Mercedes Showroom in Paris during a four-day stopover after he and my stepmother, Odette, spent a week in Geneva, where Odette's United Nations job took her twice-yearly.

Thinking about my dad makes me terribly sad. Maybe today isn't the day to wear his coat—not that I'm superstitious, because if that were the case I wouldn't be living in his old apartment. But still. I turn away from the mirror and stare into my living room, suddenly not certain at all as to why I'm not panicking, running amok, charging at walls, ramming my head into the plaster. Am I in an alternate universe, a place where Eric Robespierre doesn't have any ugly 3:00 p.m. appointment with the urologist because his PSA is just fine (thank you very much for asking)?

I think I'll check the hall closet for another coat. I'm distracted by the sunlight pouring in through my living-room windows, which face east, out into a large enclosed courtyard covered in artificial grass, where kids and adults play sports and workmen are still ripping up the pavement. The staccato thumping and whomping suddenly roars back into my consciousness—so much for an alternate universe.

Buildings identical to mine surround the courtyard, and between these red-brick boxes there's an open area that provides me with a clear view of the East River. Today the river is calm and right now free of boats and the pesky seaplanes that constantly land at the 34th Street Heliport, fourteen or so blocks north of me. The sky is also free of the traffic helicopters that can make life hell, incessantly circling, around and around, the sound of their droning motors so excruciatingly disturbing that more than once they have provoked fantasies in which I magically turn into Rambo or The Terminator, hoist an RPG to my shoulders, and shoot these noisy sons of bitches out of the sky.

I also face the FDR, a highway that runs up and down the east side of New York. Traffic is moving freely and almost soundlessly—but I'm probably used to the whooshing sound, so ordinary car engines don't register—however, the occasional Harley racing by at ninety miles an hour can rattle my bones and make me reach for the nonexistent RPG.

I begin to brew my coffee, and when the light doesn't go on I check Mr. Coffee. No water —the second time in less than a week. My mind does a walkabout when the life of my coffee maker is at risk. I add the water; I don't seem to be learning from my mistakes. I have to concentrate, but it's nearly impossible. I can't control myself—just round the corner loom sonograms and biopsies. I know about these procedures because I've been spending time on the Internet, reading up on bad walnuts.

I go online Monday afternoon, around 5:30 p.m.—I'm proud I'm able to hold off that long. Naturally, I begin thinking about going online moments after I make my urology appointment—that's a lie . . . I begin thinking about it as soon as I get the call from Lombardo, but instead make phone calls and get loaded at lunch, all failed attempts at reassuring myself nothing's really wrong. Eventually my darker angels take over and morbid curiosity gets the better of me. I'm particularly anxious to read about PSA numbers. Are mine dangerously high or just worrisome? Well, I learn lots about PSA numbers, more than I want to know; unfortunately, I don't stop there, and find myself absorbed in an introduction to bad walnuts, followed by paragraphs on screening and diagnosis, complications—complications?—hold it right there! Why do I fixate on this section and continually look for more information in this category, and not on just one site—no, not just one site, but at least a dozen more?

There's another thing that's frightening—sonograms. I didn't have to read more than a few lines to realize it's an *internal* examination. The thought of someone shoving a tube up my *tush* (*sans* drugs) sends a coldness rippling through my body, conjures up images of me writhing in pain on the examining table, gripping the table edges, moaning, maybe even screaming—because I know that if a simple prostate exam is a seven on the rectum scale of pain, tube-shoving has got to be a ten. Let me tell you, if you want to make yourself crazy, the Web is the place to go, and that is why from Monday until now the computer is dark.

I'm packing my iPod and a hardboiled Ian Rankin mystery; I anticipate a long wait in the urologist's office and I'm going to need something to distract me. I check the weather on Ten-Ten WINS New York: "You give us 22 minutes we'll give you the world." Now I'm wondering how many more twenty-two minutes I'll have.

It's chilly, so I layer up, even though I know it's going to be a pain in the ass taking the stuff off when I have to strip down to my civvies for the exam, a pain in the ass—Jesus H. Christ on a popsicle stick, what a choice of words! The charcoal-grey sweater I choose isn't particularly lucky or unlucky, so I'll wear it. Forget Pop's Mercedes leather—I have a nice blue Armani overcoat (from my spiffy ad years), still in good condition, certainly big enough to allow me to wear a sweater and sports jacket, so no layering problem, and if I bring my canvas cargo bag, I can even store the sweater if I'm too hot. The jacket is grey and blends in nicely with the jeans and sweater, not that anyone's going to see me unless I get good news from the urologist and decide to hoopla it up with a glass of *vino* at one of the fancy-dancy wine bars on Madison.

Just the notion of good news produces enough Dopamine to send the smile message shooting down my nerve pathways, but can I hold this grin? Can I continue to see myself sitting in that wine bar, sipping that twelve-dollar glass of Pinot noir out of a tall, wide-rim glass (not one of those tiny things you couldn't even gargle from), feeling A-OKAY, not even caring I'm being hosed on the wine, and could get the same glass of Pinot (all right, out of a tiny glass) in my nabe for eight bills?

I decide to walk to the subway, catch the local up to my stop, then walk the remaining few blocks to the doctor's office. Walking is a great distraction—or should be, if I pay attention to what's around me and don't zone out. I'm also taking my pocket-size digital camera, so if I decide to take a thank-God-it's-over walkabout, I can grab some shots of the famous fall foliage that makes Central Park a three-strip Technicolor wonder.

What about the wine bar? Does a walkabout mean no hoopla? Doubt dries up the Dopamine drip and my grin disappears. Just as I get to the door, I look into the hall mirror (something I rarely do) and there he is, staring at me with his grey eyes, ice cold.

"Let's dangle, pally."

Out on the street all I can think about is the sonogram, and is it really going to be as painful as I imagine? *Stop this!* At the corner of Lexington and 23rd Street, I'm caught up in a mob of college-age boys and girls going in and out of Baruch College. It's like Grand Central Station, and no easy task to cross Lex. The kids are going in all directions, weighed down with back-breaking book bags, staring straight ahead, down at the ground, or chatting up their friends in animated conversation; everyone wears headphones leading to iPods or cell phones.

I cross over to the west side of Lex and now I'm in the thick of the subway mob. As I make my way up the block, it suddenly occurs to me how easy it would be to slip into the body of one of these healthy-looking male students. They're so carefree and jubilant, they wouldn't even notice. Look at them, flirting with female classmates or just horsing around with their male buds. They wouldn't feel a thing. Look how they're smoking, eating chips and gulping sodas; supermen all, in the prime of their invincibility, cocks hard in their pants as they periodically check their packages in a show of macho behavior; in their own world and completely powerless to prevent me from using my magical powers to take over and body-snatch them.

Most are of color, with a few white boys in the mix. I'm following two in particular: Latinos who are muscular, well-built guys with enormous book bags strapped to their shoulders, the back-breaking load enough to buckle my knees and finish off my already herniated disc (between L4 and L5, to be exact). I only wish I could see what books they're reading, figure out which of the two is the smarter—but then I'm thinking, what does it matter? It'll still be me in the body—my consciousness, my smarts, my soul, my neurosis. One hundred percent intact, only I'll be forty years younger—forty years healthier—forty years, boyo—forty fucking years!

Whoops, almost got hit by a wheelchair. Keep your head up, you know better than to daydream in front of the United Cerebral Palsy building, where victims of this debilitating disease wait by the door in their motorized chairs to be ushered to one of the specially equipped yellow buses lined up at the curbside. Occasionally, one will make a beeline for a bus, unattended, completely unaware of the crowds or their handicap, and clip an unsuspecting pedestrian who's not paying attention.

Not today, Masked Man! I just dodge a young teen (attached to an oxygen tank), and make it to the subway, but I'm not completely unscathed. Suppose that was me or one of my kids in a wheelchair? Suddenly, my body-snatching fantasies are over, and I'm thanking my lucky stars I ain't worse off than I am. I'm amazed at my maturity. Unfortunately this only works for the next fifteen minutes, which is how long it takes me to get up to my stop.

The train ride is non-eventful, just the way I like it: no power failures, smoky track fires, or delays caused by police activity trapping you in hot crowded cars; no foul-smelling beggars harassing you for money; no scary toughs looking you over, licking their lips in anticipation of making you the next person they'll be carving up. I wonder if I *were* singled out by a knife-wielding nut, if I could get some sympathy if I told him I have bad walnuts, or should I act crazier—curse him and the horse he rode in on; scream, "I've got cancer! Kill me! I don't wanna live, anyway!"

Oh fuck, I said the C word! Worse, I admitted I *have* the dreaded disease. *Never, ever, say stuff like that again, even if you are playing Let's Pretend in your head. You'll give yourself the evil eye. You'll fuck yourself up!* I take it back! I take it back—but does taking it back remove the evil eye?

I get off at my stop and follow the snaking line of passengers slowly making their agonizing way off the crowded platform, single-filing it up the narrow stairway built to accommodate a third of today's riding public. Unlike everyone else, I'm in no hurry. I finally reach the street and head west. Freshly washed, chauffer-driven silver or black Bentleys, Roll Royces, Maybachs, and Mercedes limos—plus an assortment of huge, shined-up SUVs you can see your reflection in—clog the narrow streets, which are lined with majestic limestone townhouses.

I keep my ears open in case my real father, upon gazing out from his mansion, recognizes his long lost boy and heir to his enormous fortune, hurriedly pushes aside the floor-to-ceiling French windows and frantically yells, "Son! Son! Son!"

On the other hand, would I rather be back in the body of one of those healthy, young college studleys? Rich and sick? Healthy and poor? Rich and sick? Healthy and poor?

Buddha in the brain with a riddle? Mantra mind-game migraine! Mantra mind-game migraine!

I'm in a blur. *Gots to pay attention, gots to pay attention.* It's north one block, then cross the street. Okay—I'm good to go. I turn the corner and the solemnity of the weathered facade chills my bones. I don't see the doctor's name outside the main entrance, so I ask the doorman. He directs me to the small doorway a couple of steps north. I find the door and see the doctor's gold nameplate. I try the knob—the door's locked. Good sign: nobody home. I'm outta here.

Sigh. I don't think so. I ring the bell. I'm buzzed in.

"Shit and double-shit!"

I'm in Shit Lockdown again.

The large and surprisingly shabby-drab waiting room (*Come on, this is the fucking Upper East Side, for Christ's sake!*) is filled with men my age or older, each as lifeless as the décor. Some are with family, but most are by themselves like me; drained by paralyzing fright, they avoid eye contact with me and the other patients.

This is going to be real fun . . . .

There must be five very stern-looking women behind the reception desk, each wearing headsets; their brains could be in Des Moines or Mumbai, for they show absolutely no awareness of the life forms on the other side of the desk. A few are on the phone (probably telling patients they're going to die), while others bang away on computer keyboards (probably Dear Patient letters informing them they're also going to die).

No one bothers to look up when I enter. The tacky, computer-generated sign on the desk says: *Please sign in. Then wait to be called.* I attempt to make eye contact, looking for the opportunity to smile, crack a joke, fawn—anything to make them like me more than the other patients. *Bupkis*, nothing, *nada, rien.*

No muss, no fuss. I sign the registry. I'm not going to break their rules, draw their attention, screw myself to the wall. I scope out the place and see that there are rows of seats on both sides of the aisle, plus three facing me. Most are taken (this is a real happening place), but I spot two empties on my right, way down at the end. I quickly grab them, put my cargo bag on one, then stand in front of the other while removing my overcoat, jacket, and sweater. I'm sweating like a pig. The Fear. The man directly to my right doesn't even look up and acknowledge my presence. *Screw you, too, buddy boy.*

Should I keep all these clothes on the empty seat next to me, or at least hang up my overcoat on the rack across the room? I'm normally distrustful of hanging clothes up in doctors' offices because I think they'll be stolen, but I know it's really more like I can't let go of myself. See, the clothes are a symbol representing your very core being. Head pounding. Eyes popping.

Wow—Dr. Phil in the cerebral cortex with a fucking explanation for everything. Living-God migraine! Living-God migraine!

I shake my head free of the brain chatter and I go to hang up my damn coat. *Screw it! If I got bad walnuts, what more do I have to lose?* My heart's racing. Forget about the bad walnuts—just let me get the hell outta here without getting a heart attack.

I hang up the coat and stuff the sweater in my cargo bag. The jacket's a problem. I decide I'll hang it up (under the coat, for added security), but before I do I have to remove the good stuff. I could put everything into my cargo bag (like when I go through airport security), but for lengthy holds it's not an option. Only problem is keys, wallet, eyeglass, camera, phone, and iPod won't all fit in my jeans pocket. (No, I do not wear a freaking fanny pack). What to do, what to do? I'm really sweating now. Okay—camera and iPod go into cargo bag, everything else gets jammed into my jeans.

As I sit my duff down, a well dressed, carefully groomed, middle-aged gentleman, wealth and power dripping from every Italian silk thread, enters the room. I'm distracted and no longer worry about bulging pockets. Now I'm preoccupied with the newcomer, wondering why Mr. Dripping Wealth and Power isn't able to buy off bad walnuts. Perhaps that's not why he's here—perhaps illness is not part of his MO. Naturally, Mr. Dripping Wealth and Power doesn't think the rules posted on the ticky-tacky sign apply to him, so he stridently declares he's there to see Doctor So-and-so whom, he adds, is waiting to see him. *Yeah, right, that'll work.*

Naturally, he gets no response from the Headset Crowd, and I mean not even an eye twitch. On the other hand, all of us waiting-room chickens are at parade attention. So what does the idiot moron do? He leans over the desk and is one millisecond away from reaching out and tapping the Headset closest to him, but before he makes this fatal mistake, Headset's mean-bitch antennae come alive and she looks up, freezes Mr. Dripping Wealth and Power with a chilling stare that makes me shudder. He nods, stares blankly at the sign, nods again. Reluctantly, he picks up a pen and scratches out his name. I bet if he had time to think it over, he would have used his solid-gold Mont Blanc, because it's obvious he isn't used to touching, let alone writing with anything as offensive as the cheap plastic pen he awkwardly holds at arm's length. I can only see a portion of his neck, but even from my limited view I'm amazed at how veins can balloon out that much without bursting. This is one guy who might get a heart attack before me.

During this little drama, the Headsets never look up, and when it's over the rest of us return to our private hell. I don't have to tell you there's a lot of tension in this office, and I'm not feeling the love. This is going to be even worse than I thought. I realize I'm still sweating. I take out a handkerchief (thank God it's clean and pressed) and wipe down my forehead, cheeks, and neck. No one seems to notice. How can that be? I'm watching everyone, everything. Maybe this is not a good thing. I need to relax, distract myself. Staring at a roomful of sick guys is giving me the willies. Does everyone here have bad walnuts? Looks that way. I open my bag and pull out the Rankin mystery. But I can't concentrate, and unless I can muster up some manly discipline, this definitely will not be my finest hour.

Tell me, why can't they make the waiting rooms more inviting? Don't these geniuses know by creating doom-and-gloom surroundings they invite the demons in, cause patients greater apprehension that can only worsen their condition? Come on, what would it really cost these so-called healers to create patient-friendly environments? A simple color change to a soothing pale yellow would be a nice start. Add in some relaxing meditative music, perhaps the sounds of the sea. Pleasant aromatic fragrances like you get when you walk through the cosmetic sections at Saks or Bloomie's would also do the trick—help us to release Dopamine and the other restorative hormones, neurotransmitters, and brain chemicals we so desperately need as we huddle grim-faced, stomachs churning, rectums knotted, scrotums shriveled, hearts racing, the invisible, ever-threatening sword of Damocles inching closer, making the hairs on the back of our necks stand at attention.

I glance down again at my book, try to lose myself in mystery. Rankin's prose and storytelling gifts are magical, but it's not computing; all I'm seeing are individual words, disjointed, unconnected. I try reading the same page twice; maybe this will force me to focus, switch my brain on to Understanding Mode. But, no. I'm trying in vain to stop my mind from wandering to dark, fearful places it shouldn't go to when I hear a woman's voice call my name, mispronouncing it as usual.

I stand, wave at this new person who has appeared magically from God knows where. She's wearing street clothes like the Headset Women, but I think she's special. She's Eric's guide, taking me across the River Styx! No—the last time I looked my name was Robespierre, not Odysseus. I stand to make sure she realizes I'm here and won't mistakenly skip over me like the counter guys at Ess-A-Bagel do on Sunday morning when you don't yell loud enough for them when they call your number. At Ess-A-Bagel I yell, "Yo" (the place is full of yuppies, and that's what they yell), but this is a more formal environment, so I shout out, "Here!" just like I did in school. In case anyone should come in and need a seat, I remove my cargo bag from the adjoining chair and place it on the one I'm vacating. Still no acknowledgement from the guy next to me—

What? I'm Mr. Fucking Cellophane Man? I turn and head for the unknown. No one else looks up or gives a good goddamn. Maybe I *am* invisible?

I quickly approach the desk. Guide Woman—unsmiling, unwelcoming—wants to know what doctor I'm seeing and if I'm a new patient.

Look, you moron of an idiot—I wrote it down on the sign-up sheet! Big smile now, Eric, me boyo.

"I'm here to see Dr. Upper East Side, and I'm a first-time patient."

I'm glad last night I slept with a hanger in my mouth, stretched it out so I'm smiling like The Joker, 'cause Jack's in the house now.

Moron-of-an-idiot, I'm going to make you love me. Bigger, wider smile.

"What insurance do you have?"

Well, that didn't work—then again, who knows how much more disinterested she'd be if I hadn't tried a smile? Maybe it's not in her personality to be friendly? Perhaps "has to be tepid, half-hearted, show disinterest" is part of her job description, or does she do it to survive? Let's be real now: how many guys with bad walnuts do you have to make nicey-nice to before you go Loony-Tunes and need a rubber room? The ACDC song pops into my head, only I'm changing the lyrics.

"I've got bad walnuts

I've got bad walnuts

And they're such bad walnuts

Dirty bad walnuts

And he's got bad walnuts,

And he's got bad walnuts,

But we've got the baddest walnuts of them all!"

They should be playing the song over loudspeakers, don't you think?

"Medicare and AARP," I reply.

Half-hearted Guide Woman is talking, informing me she's going to need my insurance cards and that I'll have to fill out some patient-information forms. She fishes under the desk for the necessary papers, then in her lackadaisical manner pushes them across the desktop. God forbid she should exert herself, maybe break a goddamn nail—which could use some polish, by the way. Something colorful, not drab like her and this damn office; maybe put a little spark in her day and mine.

"Okay," I agree, still smiling into her eyes, still trying to make her love me. *Bupkis*, nothing, *nada, rien.* I nod, quickly pull out my wallet, remove the insurance cards, reluctantly hand them over. I might have grown a larger set of balls when I hung up my coat, but they're not *that* big; nope, I'm still a Nervous Nelly who irrationally believes the odds are more than even money this lady will lose the cards from here to the copying machine. Lucky for me she doesn't go more than two feet, giving me a clear shot at her the entire time. I'm so worried about the umbilical cord being severed I don't think to question how much of the bill will be covered, never even consider the possibility there will be "exceptions" (i.e. ways to screw policyholders) and I'll be on the hook for money I don't have. *Stupid me.* My hands are in the ready position when she returns, her head angled slightly to the left, eyes already distracted, concentrating on how to tune out the next victim.

I am Siamese—no eye contact, if you please.

I trudge back to my seat. Two more worn-out souls enter; I'm relieved I'm not hogging a second seat. Only—stranger than strange—they don't look for a resting place, but instead—their eyes front, gait shuffling slow—they reach the front desk, stand side by side, shoulder to shoulder, like planes docking at their respective gates. It doesn't make sense. Don't they know the right move would be to grab a seat, then go up and sign in? But . . . didn't I do the same thing? Yeah—well—this is my first time, so I don't know the lay of the land, but I get the vibe from their beaten-down faces these guys are regs, know wait time is twenty-to-thirty minutes, should be thinking, *Seat first, sign in second.*

Just as I sit myself down, another Guide Babe, only this one is dressed in white, appears and calls out a name. Is she the one?

A spoon is not a spoon; *Keanu is now in the house.* A concrete block dressed as a man in a well-worn dark suit bursting at the buttons, white open-neck shirt, about forty, days' growth of hair blackening his olive-complected cheeks, slowly rises from his seat against the far wall, and bellows in a thick Russian accent the correct pronunciation of his name.

Wow, does this guy got a set. Obviously the Russian Bear doesn't know the score, thinks his KBG tough-guy routine will frighten the staff the way it did when he tossed some poor soul into a cell at Lubyanka.

Mind your own beeswax. I quickly fill in name, address, etc., etc., then come to twenty or so questions relating to various illnesses and medical conditions, all of which I don't have. After answering no to every single question, the thought occurs to me that I shouldn't be here, because I'm one healthy son of a bitch and all that can happen here is they can make me sick and die. I think about leaving. The door is only two feet away. No one would notice. No one would care. I visualize myself walking through Central Park, the millstone flung into the bushes, a buoyancy returning to my step. I smile at everyone I see. They smile back. I've even lost twenty pounds. It's a beautiful vision—a glorious three-strip Technicolor life.

The last two sheets are release forms. I sign each without reading them. I know they deal with being responsible for paying your bills and for indemnifying the doctor should you get sick, die, or suffer the ill effects of his indifference in the next fifty years, regardless of if he treats you or not. I have no choice. Sign, or get the fuck out. (That is a corollary to *Take the medicine or die*.)

I look up. It's now standing-room only, even though the seat to right of me is still vacant. What's with that? Do I smell? That's crazy—even if I do (which I don't), none of these new guys ever get close enough to find out. The newbies run the gamut in color from simply nervous-pale to ashen-grave, from the physically fit to the wobbly. Where am I in this mix? Do I see myself the way others see me? If they would look—which they don't. What's with that? Why won't anyone else look another person in the eye? What are they afraid of? If someone were to catch my eye, I'd nod—soldier to soldier, joined forever in our battle against the bad walnut.

Marlowe turns his granite jaw ever so slightly in my direction. My pal's just taken the seat on my right. I nod. He nods, his eyes totally obscured by the brim of his fedora. I'm not alone anymore. I stuff the Rankin book back into my cargo bag; notice the author's photo. Damn—he's young and healthy, too. But no way I can body snatch from a photo.

I hear a call for "Raspberries," and since the last time I looked this was a doctor's office and not a fruit stand, I assume the nurse who's emerged from a connecting hallway to scan our lifeless faces is calling my name. She's the one! There is no spoon! I stand.

Goodbye, Keanu—Kirk is in now the house.

"I'm Eric Robespierre."

I'm expecting the others to stand and one by one shout: "I'm Eric Robespierre!" "I'm Eric Robespierre!" "I'm Eric Robespierre!" The trouble is, I'm not Kirk Douglas, and this isn't *Spartacus*. No one moves, much less utters a single syllable to save me.

They're my bad walnuts—I'm on my own!

As if mesmerized, I follow my guide's swaying body parts—*swish-swish, sway-sway*. I get it, I understand what these pecker-pokers are up to—showing me this lovely *tush* so I can get it up this one last time before they turn me into a eunuch. It's urology's version of the condemned man's last meal. Nice.

I'm walking though a maze of corridors, passing examining rooms and book-lined offices. A mob of doctors, nurses, technicians (who can tell one from another?) moves in and out of my path. I stop counting at ten. Which one is mine? I smile at every single one, but none bother to even glance my way and return my salutation. This wouldn't happen if I were a rock star, politico, or The Donald, safely cocooned by security goons wearing aviator glasses, tiny earpieces, and packing SIG Sauer P229s.

I make up a joke. *What do you call a group of security guards in a pecker-poker's office? Gorillas in the piss . . . Heh, heh, heh . . .* I'm picking up an alcohol smell . . . or something worse? The Fear! Me! I am The Fear. The Fear is me at this exact moment in time, moving dreamlike slow through an unfamiliar, antiseptic maze. Not Ira, Michael Milken, Mayor Giuliani, Robert DeNiro, a made-up character in one of my stories—me—me—The Fear . . . moving toward what?

I'm led directly into Dr. Upper East Side's office. The first thing I notice is how professorial (i.e. fucking smart) this guy looks, and when he greets me with a thick Teutonic accent the deal is sealed. Dr. Upper East Side obviously comes from the land of Krupp, Braun, Messerschmitt, and Mercedes Benz; if there is a race of more obsessively thorough and detail-orientated people, clue me in. Oh, they can be fallible. Werner Von Braun, for one—who claimed he aimed for the stars, but instead hit London. Those V-2s were the shit, weren't they?

When Dr. Upper East Side stands to greet me, firmly shaking my hand, I get the sense that beneath his long, white coat—immaculately starched and wrinkle free—lies a rock-hard, six-pack-abs bod.

"Mr. Robespierre."

He correctly pronounces my name. Would you expect less? He jokes about my infamous ancestor and hopes he won't suffer a similar fate under my hands. He smiles. Is this a joke, a threat–what? I smile. Right back at ya.

Then I speak:

"I hope so, too."

He grins. Something bad is coming thisaway. Can't be an anti-Semitic thing going on here, not with my name, not if he knows old Maximilian was born a Catholic. Then, again he's The Man; has special urological gifts; most likely can see through my pants and read *Jude* where the foreskin once lived, a tell-tale giveaway I'm not related to the frog revolutionary.

Curiously, as if he also has the powers of mind reading, he asks for my history. I'm dazzled; then I realize—*Idiot, he doesn't mean my lineage. He's interested in my medical history.* I start from Dr. Lombardo's phone call. I try to be thorough, coldly clinical, and show off how smart I am. He writes everything down. Then he starts with the questions.

"Do you have any trouble urinating? Do you have a strong stream? Do you experience any burning sensation when urinating? Any pain when you urinate? How about at night—how often do you get up to urinate?"

He's gentle and kind in manner, but I'm seeing the cunning Major Strasser in his house. So who's in mine—Rick or Victor Laszlo?

I answer assuredly in the negatory, my tone and body language drawing the natural conclusion: no symptoms equals no bad walnuts? (I'm now Bogie's Rick.)

What the hell is he writing? My answers are short and sweet. It shouldn't take him this long to jot them down, unless—unless what? Could he be multi-tasking? Writing someone else's report? Maybe something personal: a love letter; article for a medical journal; how about a book, a murder mystery, screenplay. Everyone's writing a screenplay, and his deals with uncovering Nazi gold. *Come on, can't you be more original? An* arms dealer? I have it! Crystal-meth manufacturer, and for a backstory a cheating wife?

"Mr. Robespierre, please follow me into the examining room. We will require some blood, administer a sonogram, have you provide a urine sample, and then we'll come back and talk about next steps."

Next steps, that's a good sign that implies a future. He stands. He seems even more imposing than when I entered. Maybe that's because I'm still sitting. I rise to my feet, surprised to find that I'm not shaking or wobbling. I follow him like a little dog trotting after his master. He's going to examine my prostate. I'm ready for a little discomfort, at the worst a little pain, but he's probably done a thousand finger jobs, so it should be painless. Right? Right! It's the other thing—the snake-a-tube-up-your-ass sonogram—I'm scared to death of.

Just before I enter the small examining room, I see Marlowe come toward me, smile, and swiftly brush by, eyebrows twitching, grey eyes twinkling imperceptibly under his grey fedora—unnoticeable to the untrained eye, unseen by anyone but me. I nod and take courage in his presence. I take a deep breath; say, *Fuck it,* to myself; and enter the small, white-walled room.

"Mr. Robespierre, please remove your shoes, pull down your trousers to your knees, your drawers halfway, and then get up on the examining table."

Long gone are the flexible days when I can easily bend and remove my shoes, so I take a seat and get the job done the old-fogey way. I see I've brought my cargo bag; this is a good thing. Unfortunately, I don't remember bringing it with me when I left the waiting room; this is a bad thing. I look out into the hallway as a nurse passes. I see a silhouette on the wall: a hand tipping the brim of a fedora as the shadowy figure moves aside to let the nurse pass in the narrow corridor. I smile, stick my sneakers under the chair, and stand. The table is low enough for me to push myself up onto it without using the footrest. I do it confidently, as smoothly as any gymnast, happily dangling my feet when a little gas uncontrollably escapes—thank God without sound, but suddenly two new fears unleash the adrenaline flow: 1) I haven't thoroughly cleaned myself out, or 2) I will become incontinent. I break out in a swamp of sweat.

The doctor half-turns his back to me, but I can still see him putting a latex glove on his right hand. I quickly pull down my pants and boxer shorts, dark ones chosen so no stains will show up. He turns and approaches. *Dum-de-dum-dum.*

"Mr. Robespierre, would you lie down and then turn to your left?"

Brain freeze! Left or right? I trust my instincts, turn toward the wall.

"Just relax," he says.

His heavy accent no longer reminds me of Conrad Veidt's Colonel Strasser, but now Otto Preminger, when he played Colonel von Scherbach, the camp commandant in *Stalag 17*. Naturally, I'm no longer Rick, but Sefton, the William Holden character: sardonic, cagy, and casually non-caring. Holden's my favorite non-noir actor, and as Joe Gillis—the equally sardonic loser screenwriter in *Sunset Boulevard*—gives his best performance. It's an identity I have assumed many times, but I'm not in my screenwriting role now. I'm in 'Escape Examining Room 17' mode. I'm Sefton—and I'm getting out of here alive.

"Ooh-ouch, this hurts!"

I'm out of character as soon as I feel sharp hard nails digging into my soft, unforgiving tissue. You would think someone who does this examination for a living would trim his goddamn nails!

He pokes, grips, feels, fingers, while I'm seeing horrifying images of my tiny walnut in the grips of a madman planning his wife's murder, grabbing her fortune and buying more crystal meth, and—just like that—the examination is over.

"Mr. Robespierre, I don't find your prostate to be enlarged or misshaped in anyway."

I nod and smile dumbly. "Misshaped" is code for tumors bulging out; I know this because I read it on the Internet. Okay, I ducked *that* bullet. How many more to go?

Dr. Upper East Side removes his latex glove and tosses it into a metal waste receptacle.

"Mr. Robespierre, please lie back and keep your drawers down."

He moves in front of a tan-colored machine, adjusts some dials, turns the screen on, and finally picks up a similarly colored wand. The words "ultrasound machine" flash in Las Vegas neon across my brain.

Whoop-dee-do! My heart's jumping out of my chest with joy. Unless he's going to stick that wand down my throat, this is going to be an external examination!

"Mr. Robespierre, please lie still."

What's with this "Mr. Robespierre"? Why does he have to keep calling me by my surname every two minutes? Is he checking to make sure he's examining the right patient? Maybe one time he cut off a testicle when he should have been biopsying a walnut? At first my eyes are closed, but now I cautiously open them, and, without moving my head, strain my peepers upward so I can see the screen. Without thinking of the consequences, I stare at images of my lower abdomen or what I guess is my lower abdomen. Dr. Upper East Side slowly, expertly moves the magic wand. I see masses pulsate and undulate, as if suspended in liquid, moving slowly in rhythm to the vagaries of the solution. How can that be possible? The wand gradually travels north and south, then east and west. I feel a slight coldness as the plastic tip presses gently on my flesh. White masses, dark shadows, then dark masses and white shadows, none of it recognizable, all of it very much alive—all of it in me.

I suddenly remember a similar screen, but the circumstances are so completely different that I nearly don't make the connection. It's when my ex is pregnant with our first and then with our second, when the ob-gyn proudly shows us our child's embryo and we see its beating heart. I run the film of those sacred events over in my brain and the images fill me with joy, but it's only momentary. I need to look away, shut my eyes as the embryos turn into cancer cells.

I open and close my eyes. Why do I see bad walnuts where there are none? I'm a nut job, that's why. I should have paid more attention to those tumor photos. I didn't; I couldn't muster the courage. Fear may be the mind-killer, but ignorance is bliss. Everything's a fucking trade-off, isn't it?

He's going to take my blood himself? This I don't believe. What a nice, caring guy. Then I think, maybe he doesn't rate a nurse? How could that be? No money? Is he being sued for malpractice? They don't like him? He gropes them? The doctor gently presses his fingers into my flesh, palpates the veins in my left arm, then my right, finally choosing one in my left arm. My brain's obviously in Shit Lockdown, because I've completely forgotten about my rolling veins and I have no idea why he's choosing one arm over another. I don't feel the needle going in, and tell him so. Oh, I got it: He does everything himself, because he knows no one can do it better. I nod, manage a weak smile, turn away. Never, ever, look at what they're doing, especially when they're drawing blood.

The first time I went to Dr. Lombardo I broke this rule, because I wanted to impress his nurse with my macho-macho. Instead I nearly panicked and pulled out the needle, because after she filled up the first vial, she filled another, then finally a third. You tell me, what does she need three vials for? Another thing— the color, it was scary dark, crimson, really, and that frightened me. Not that I know the color of healthy blood, but when I nick myself shaving or give myself a paper cut it's usually much brighter, so naturally I'm thinking I have a blood disease and that further scares the bejesus out of me. *Get a grip*, I say, but then I figure, *Three vials, damn, I'm going to get faint, pass out, because three vials ain't shit.* Suddenly it's over, and Lombardo's nurse is asking me to press hard on the tiny piece of cotton while she gets a Band-Aid, then she's covering the tiny puncture— only it's HIM asking me to press hard. *Yes, mein Führer!*

He gives me a Svengali stare. Oh shit, he reads minds! Think of something else—distract, sidetrack, confuse: *That was painless. Thank you, doctor.*

He nods, secures the cotton with a Band-Aid. I want to reach out and grip his shoulders, convince him the Führer thing is just Jewish Comic Relief—"shtetl shtick," embedded in the defense-mechanism code of my tribe's DNA. I want to demonstrate, in no uncertain terms, how happy I am he's my doctor, tell him how much I value his expertise, how I'm ready to put my life in his caring, all-healing hands. But I don't say a word—he's talking.

He meticulously tears off the electronic printout, gently pushes the ultrasound machine away from the table. Oh great, *Siemens*—the machine is manufactured by Siemens; this beats the fucking band!

FYI, Siemens supported the Hitler regime, contributed to the war effort, and participated in the "Nazification" of the economy, having many factories in and around notorious extermination camps such as Auschwitz and using slave labor from concentration camps to build electric switches for military uses. There's more, but these are the salient points that pop into my head.

How come I know so much about Siemens, you ask? Well, it just so happens that yesterday, while browsing the Internet in my continuing, but cautious researching (I say *cautious* because you want to avoid anything too graphic that will really frighten your ass), info on sonograms and ultrasound equipment leads me to the Siemens's page on Wikipedia. Coincidence? I think not!

"Mr. Robespierre, please get dressed, then go into the adjoining bathroom and provide a urine sample, and when you are finished, come into my office."

He Svengalis me again; when that doesn't provoke a response (*what?—he thinks I'm going to click heels and give him a "Sieg Heil"?*), he throws me another something-bad-is-coming-this-way smile.

You know what, sports fans? I don't give a shit. *No tubes up the ass today, Herr Doktor—no tubes up the ass today!*

"Not a problem," I murmur meekly, and with that he's gone.

I look down at my drawers. How can I get dressed when I'm using my right hand to press down on the cotton ball while my left arm is extended out? More to the point, how can I face him again if he thinks I think he's Der Führer? Another thing, did he tell me how long I have to press down on the cotton, a ball much larger than the one Lombardo applied?

Well, at least he's not skimping on the supplies, and by the looks of it, he didn't jack me on the ultrasound. Then again, I don't know how long these exams are supposed to last, how much electricity they're supposed to use, stuff like that; screwing patients on Medicare is definitely on the brain. Why wouldn't it be, after Google brought me to page after page detailing how doctors treat Medicare patients like second-class citizens because they're pissed the government doesn't adequately reimburse them? (But now does this make sense, when secondary insurance is supposed to cover the difference?)

Did he say five minutes? I think he did say that, but my mind is six ways to Sunday and I'm not paying attention. *Shit Lockdown. Shit Lockdown.* I have to be more careful, can't let my mind do dangerous walkabouts like this.

I split the difference: using one one-hundreds, I count two and a half minutes to myself. I lose count twice, but don't start over, although I do consider the option. When I'm finished, I quickly dress, then make my way into the bathroom. Whoa, Nelly! A tall stack of empty vials, pyramidal in shape, dominates the little room, and appears ready to topple should someone pull out a cup from anywhere but the very top—something someone might very well do if the urge to pee is so overwhelming that letting the one-eyed snake out must come first and filling up second (in mid-stream, holding on with one hand while the other reaches out for any vial before you pee out).

On another similar, but smaller shelf is space for filled vials. In case you left your detection skills at the door, there are typed signs telling you where to fill up and where to drop off. I'm hearing "Walk Like An Egyptian" in my head, but no dancing today—there isn't enough room.

I usually have a problem peeing on demand, but—surprise, surprise—I'm in control of my nerves and, like a good soldier, follow orders quickly. Filling these little devils is always tricky; first off, how much is enough? I try to go three-quarters, but I'm never able to do it without stopping and starting: sometimes over-filling—messy-messy—sometimes going under and discovering I'm unable to start again. And understand this is under normal circumstances, never when bad walnuts are in the mix.

Oh great, a weak stream, starting, stopping, starting and stopping—like I don't want to give it up. But finally, I'm finished. I put the vial down. I've missed something; the pens! Oh, shit! I grab one, pick up the vial, make sure the cap is tight, write my name on the sticker wrapped around its center—not my full name, only room for "Robespierre," and then only if I make the letters tiny and run the last three off the line.

I never realized how hot my pee is. I carefully place the warm cup down on the counter top, squirt a little bit of soap onto my hands, wash thoroughly, and dry them with a towel. I do a thousand-mile stare into the mirror, wondering if tomorrow's pee will have the smell of bad walnuts.

I leave, and in half a dozen steps I'm in his office, catching sight of doctors and nurses crisscrossing to the left and right and, down at the end of the hall, a figure wearing a fedora. Where the hell is HE going?

I sit. Dr. Upper East Side is totally engrossed in reading the results of my ultrasound and doesn't so much as acknowledge my entrance. I know he knows I'm there; Svengali knows everything. I take the opportunity to seriously study the bookshelves lined with color-coordinated medical books, walls of degrees, awards and framed news clippings. Forget the German crap, this is The Man. He is The Shit. This reassures me. He will save me.

"Mr. Robespierre, I don't see any abnormalities here."

He raises the ultrasound readout long enough to emphasize his point, then he gently places it back down on the desk. I'm seeing this in slow-mo. I must be breathing in slow-mo, too, because I let out a sigh of relief in sync to the paper drop. He Svengalis me with those piercing, questioning eyes. Will he continue? Only the Svengali knows.

The answer comes with a clearing of the throat. The eyes soften just a touch. I'm getting a kindly professorial look now. Oh boy, is this going to be a lecture on death and dying? Nope. It's a lecture, but not the one I neurotically anticipate; instead, I'm going to be treated to a thorough description of the workings of the walnut. To make sure I clearly understand his every word, Dr. Upper East Side uses simple drawings to methodically illustrate his talk. I try to soak in each syllable, never taking my eye off his pointy finger. I really do try—I swear—but I can't help the fact my mind momentarily wanders this way and that. At first I'm thinking, *I'm a first-year med student, and isn't this cool, and won't my parents be happy when I come home in my scrubs.* Then I'm thinking, *Do first-year med students wear scrubs?* Then I'm back, locked in and focused on the urethra or is it the ureter. Then it's my father walking out of the urologist's office.

The explanation is certainly comprehensive, and offered in such an uncomplicated and straightforward way—suddenly Jack and Tom are in the house.

"I run my unit how I run my unit. You want to investigate me? Roll the dice and take your chances. I eat breakfast three-hundred yards from four-thousand Cubans who are trained to kill me, so don't think for one second that you can come down here, flash your badge, and make me nervous. Are you clear on that, Lieutenant?"

"Crystal . . . !"

Crystal . . . I stare at Dr. Upper East Side. I'm off Gitmo, back on the Upper East Side. The words *anatomy, symptoms, disease* appear—clear—appear to me—crystal clear — just as they appear to the fucked and dying when they poke trembling fingers into the alphabet soup and arrange the little white letters, one noodle making sense of another. It's their last meal and The Maker's last little joke.

"Other than a rising PSA, you are not showing any of these symptoms; therefore, the elevation may be due to an infection . . . "

Huh? What? Where the hell am I? Infection! Did he say infection? I want to jump up, pump my fist in the air and give a Marv Albert YES, but I don't move, not even an inch. I'm amazed at my self-control. He's still talking. What is he saying now? What is he doing?

"Have you ever taken Cipro?"

"No—never." I shake my head for emphasis.

Cipro . . . My euphoria is short lived. Cipro . . . This is one hell of a powerful drug, with frightening side effects.

Most Americans, including me, had never even heard of the drug until right after 9/11, when some nut job sent anthrax-laced letters to an assortment of politicos and media hot shots; then TV and print pundits were all over it. We learned that if you had shown symptoms or you had been exposed to the white powder (and I don't mean coke), Cipro was the only thing that would save your sorry ass—and even then the odds weren't so great. If that wasn't scary enough, we learned that if terrorists had decided to put this stuff into commercial and residential airshafts or general mailings like phone bills and shopper stuffers, there wouldn't have been enough Cip to give Anthrax the slip.

Naturally, panic ensued. Thankfully, most physicians acted responsibly and said no to fraidy-cat patients who wanted to hoard the drug, prompting any Nervous Nelly with the right connections to use foreign sources to illegally obtain it. Some of my friends had chosen this route and warned me that I was taking a real risk by not self-medicating, but I was more frightened by TV pundits who paraded their apocalyptic analysis of side effects than the chance I might have sat on an infected toilet seat. I may be nuts, but I'm not THAT nuts.

Dr. Upper East Side hands me the prescription.

"This is pretty strong stuff," I say.

What I really want to say is, "I'm not taking this shit—give me something that won't fucking kill me." He doesn't respond. Maybe he *can't* read my mind?

"I want you to take one in the morning and one at night for two weeks; then we'll give you another PSA. If the numbers don't go down, or they continue to go up, I'm going to insist on a biopsy."

I let this terrible news slip under a fold in my cerebellum, where it can hide until fucking doomsday. If you think I'm going to take that scenario seriously, you're out of your mind. I mutter something like, "Is there another drug you can give me for this?"

Actually, I don't think I say anything. Instead, I continue to silently seep sweat and look extremely agitated. Svengali stares at me—cold blue eyes dulled over, covered in a thin filmy coat of disgust—then his lids flutter close. Mind reader or not, I know he loathes me for doubting him.

I can see I've made an irrevocably terrible mistake. This is someone not used to being questioned. I'll bet even the IRS backs off from this guy.

Don't ever question the doctor, and always pay him before you leave the office. I can clearly hear my mother's cautionary litany, part of it anyway. How did the rest of it go? *Don't ever use a public toilet* (she wasn't talking about urinals); *take a sweater with you to the movie theater; never question the doctor, and always pay him on time.* Instructions that, up until now, have kept me from getting a venereal disease, prevented pneumonia, and successfully avoided a razor-sharp scalpel in the eye.

Dr. Upper East Side rises up from his chair so smoothly and gracefully I hardly notice the effort. I gaze up at this monstrously menacing figure, more frightening than before—or am I just hallucinating? I think loss of blood will do that to you. He glides around the desk, slickly takes my hand, and shakes it firmly, while reminding me to return for another blood test after finishing the Cipro. There will be no need to see him or make an appointment, "Just tell Reception you're my patient and you're there to have a PSA test."

His hand is warm, his palm dry. I'm cold and clammy.

He smiles. Is this supposed to mean everything is A-okay? Well, it's not. My mind is a blank. I suppose there are questions I should be asking, but my wires are frozen. I'm brain dead. *Shit Lockdown.*

I nod weakly. If I expect him to click his heels and bow to me the way James Mason did twenty-some years ago, that ain't gonna happen. What a great moment that was.

I'm with Robert Leung, my very talented art director and great friend, and we're in a cab going down Park. The cab stops at the corner of 50th and there HE is—standing there, all by himself, waiting to cross, probably heading to the Waldorf. I do a double take. Yep, it's James Mason. He's wearing a full-length, brown leather trench coat, just like the one he wears when he plays Rommel in The Desert Fox. *This is really freaky. Could it be the same one? Nah. If memory serves, that one is black. . . .* Idiot! The film is black and white*! Naturally, when coming face to face (almost) with a screen legend (*Odd Man Out, A Star is Born, Five Fingers, Lolita *and—who can forget—*Mandingo*), I act like a silly, star-struck juvenile and yell out the open window: "Mr. Mason—you're a great actor!" Boy, Eric, talk about a lack of self-control. Well, I guess flattery will get you anywhere. Graciously he gives me what I want—a James Mason performance. He smiles, raises his hand in a salute, then quickly clicks his heels and takes a deep bow. I want to leap out of the cab, only it begins to move, so I do the next best thing, stick my head out the window and wave madly. He straightens up, turns, returns my wave; I'm having heart palpitations just thinking about it.*

I now feel the Herr Doktor's hand on my left shoulder, gently guiding me out into the hallway, directing me to the left, toward the exit I imagine. Out of the corner of my eye I see him turn and head in the opposite direction. I follow the yellow brick road out of town, momentarily pausing at the front desk in case they want to stop me for some reason, like signing a form—or maybe a kind word? What dream am I living in?

I find my clothes haven't been stolen. I put my cargo bag down, slowly put on my jacket, then my overcoat. I'm careful not to make eye contact with anyone, although I have to confess I sneak a peek at several newcomers: two men half my age, both looking ghostly pale and sickly. I don't even want to imagine what they have. I just want to take in a lung full of fresh Central Park air; trot up tree-lined hills; snap off sprints in the grass; do an Ansel Adams with the digital; finally find a rock and put this shit under it.

Infection, bye-bye—happy-happy—rosy-rosy—little precious pee-pee.

I carefully transfer my wallet into my inside jacket pocket, then remove cell, iPod, and camera. I stuff the first two in the left pocket, camera into the right—knowing that in five minutes I will involuntarily check pockets, predictably going into the wrong one first, then suffer a momentary bout of panic until I discover nothing's missing. This checking business is something recent, disturbing, a warning of the coming dementia or simply inevitable stress, unavoidable when self-inflicted by a tortured tangle of brain cells.

I'm just about to leave when I suddenly get a flash of insight.

I walk back to the reception area. No one looks up. I count seven Headsets, all well trained in the art of not giving a shit. I'm standing right in front of my photocopy pal, so I figure since we have a history she'll feel the connection and look up—not in this lifetime. I throw the harridan my Superman-X-ray-vision-into-the-brain look while I silently say to her: *Look at me, look at me, LOOK AT ME.* Nothing. There's only one Svengali in her life, and it ain't me. Boy, would I love to get hold of this guy's mind-control program.

Only one thing left. I throw the bitch a Ronda *Phlegming* clearing of the throat—two, actually—in rapid-fire, machine-gun bursts. Without moving her head, or any other part of her upper body, she slowly gazes in my direction—a trick I've tried, but never mastered, because the eyestrain was too painful.

Before I wither under her gaze, I throw her my biggest smile, and say ever so obsequiously, "I'm really sorry to disturb you, but I forgot to ask Dr. Upper East Side when my PSA results will be back." Nothing . . . No response . . . Does she suddenly not speak English? "I want to make sure he has my cell so if I'm not home he can reach me."

"What's your doctor's name?"

Are you an idiot, moron? I just told you. Even more obsequiously, and with an even broader smile (one that threatens to throw my jaw out of whack), murmur, "Oh, I'm sorry—Dr. Upper East Side."

"Dr. Upper East Side never calls patients." She moves her head. Thank God. Her orbs are starting to bug out; the last thing I want is them exploding in my face—messy, messy.

"Dr. Upper East Side dictates the results, and then he sends it off to a typing service, gets it back, signs it, and mails it to you."

I'm dazed and confused; then dumbfounded; finally, disgusted. This is lawyerly cover-my-ass bullshit, rubber-stamped crap from inhuman bureaucrats, not doctor speak—not from MY doctor, not a doctor dealing with bad walnuts—MY bad walnuts.

"How long does this usually take?"

She stares at me. Do I detect a smile? "Two weeks . . . "

Central Park, in the shadows of limestone Fifth Avenue, is really something to behold, and God knows I try hard to be in the moment; and there are moments, some lasting as long as five minutes, when I do leave my worries under the nearest rock. I would have to be totally dead not to feel invigorated by the cool breeze reddening up my cheeks; blind to the palettes of luxuriating fall colors fluttering in the late afternoon glimmer. Don't think I don't try all my mind games; recite the timeworn *Carpe diem, memento mori*; smell the cappuccino (easy to do, with Starbucks on every street); and smell the roses for all the tea drinkers in the world—just to stay in the moment, tell yourself, *Nothing is promised and all you have is the here and now and here and now there are no bad walnuts. On the other hand, you do have muggings. Want to worry about something? Worry about getting your head bashed in. . . . What a time to give up sniffing glue!*

This makes me laugh. I should go out and rent *Airplane,* or maybe go to a hobby shop and buy some. The Lenny Bruce sniffing airplane glue bit comes into my head.

"Hello, sir, nice store you got here.

Gimme two weeks worth of pencils . . .

A big-boy tablet . . .

Ah—

Handful of juju beans. . .

A Webber Simpson's comic book . . .

And—ah—

Two thousand packs of airplane glue."

I'm smiling. Go home, pour yourself a large glass of *vino*, put on Lenny, Richard, Mel, and Carl—listen to every comic album you have and just forgetaboutit.

This sounds like a plan. Here's another—stay in the park until 59th Street, take a boatload of pictures, and just FORGETABOUTIT. Okay? Okay!

ROUND 2

I'M staring at the unopened vial of Cipro. It's been like this every morning since Wednesday afternoon, when I dropped fifty-six big ones over at Duane Reade—and that's WITH Medicare and the AARP discount drug plans. At these prices you would think I would be eager to gobble them down, right? *Wrong, Masked Man!*

I've come to the disturbing realization that I must have been sleeping the day they changed the good old-fashioned drugstore to mega-pharmacy—going from cozy to warehouse impersonal, from affordable to break-the-fucking-bank expensive. Perhaps if I had paid attention, this entire process wouldn't be so demoralizing.

I'm not stupid. I know conjuring up the comfy past is grabbing at the rationalization straw and sucking up the waters of excuse, but when you're staring down a vial of Cipro, afraid to take a dose because of the side effects—even more frightened that if you do and the drug doesn't bring down your PSA, then . . . then . . . —the past is a very comfortable place to be.

In case you're too young to remember what it's like to fill a prescription in a neighborhood drugstore, I'll fill you in (no pun intended). You enter, and guess what—you can actually see the entire store from the entrance! A little doorbell tingles, alerting the pharmacist (in my case, Mel), who immediately looks up and waves. I wave back.

"Hi, Eric!"

"Hi, Mel!"

Mel has owned the store since I was knee-high to a cockroach (no grasshoppers where I lived). I hand him the small square of paper with the unintelligible writing. He pulls his glasses down, stares at the script, looks up, stares at me for a minute. He's checking me out, you see, making sure my doctor (who happens to also be *his* doctor) makes the right the diagnosis. Then Mel nods, says, "It'll be a couple a minutes, so why don't you go get a soda or some candy? Tell Laura" (his wife and cashier) "it's on me."

Later we schmooze sports, talk politics, complain about the weather; before you know it I'm out the door, maybe a little gassy (I get that way when I drink carbonated stuff too fast), but otherwise, legs still strong, psyche still intact. Oh, I forgot—the whole thing's five, ten dollars tops.

All right, this is before computers, HMOs and a nation gone wild on drugs; a time when the only chain store in the nabe is the five-and-ten, known to grownups as Woolworth's. Now it's chainsaws on every block; megamaniacal merchants who need to see their names flashing in numbers equal to street-crossing signs, cutting down the mom and pop store into a bloody pulp; a deforestation as devastating to biodiversity as those taking place in Brazil and Indonesia. Mel's place is the first to feel the grim reaper, driven out of business by a company stocked with a phalanx of pharmacists and buffered by a wall of pharmacy associates who take, pass, and serve it up. Nobody ever knows their names, not that it matters—these anonymous beings change with the weather. And forget about schmoozing, unless you know how to say, "How 'bout dem Mets?" in Hindi, Farsi or Korean—that's supposing you could manage to get their attention for more than thirty seconds. Don't get me wrong, these folks are smart and they're fluent in English, but it's business English only. Oh, and did I mention how these chains started off by low-balling the little guy out of business, and now, when they own the world, charge me fifty-six bucks for Cipro?

I don't like lines, nobody does, but in New York it's a fact of life, so I can normally handle the wait. I bring a book or iPod to the post office, movie theater, even the library—where checking out can take the better part of my youth—and, of course, the pharmacy. The only time I get my nose out of joint at Duane Reade is when I've got a bad cold—then Jason's in the house and it's Friday the 13th at the pharmacy. I want my decongestants, my cough suppressants, my antibiotics, so I can crawl into my nice warm bed, pull the soft cotton covers over my aching keppe and suck my thumbee—and I want them NOW!

I never give a second thought to the people I see at the pharmacy: mostly older, mostly in poor health, clutching multiple scripts and vials, suffering from long-term illnesses like heart disease and cancer. They're invisible non-entities certainly having no relevance to my precious health or, heaven forbid, threatening my own mortality, unless I hear their chest rattling cough and immediately think *TB*. That is, until last Wednesday afternoon after I see Herr Doktor, when I go shopping for Cipro, the day reality begins to circle the drain.

Full of piss and vinegar, I get off the subway and walk straight down to 23rd Street to my Duane Reade of choice—one of five in the neighborhood, but for some reason my favorite. During my walk in Central Park I convince myself that I do not have bad walnuts. I convince myself that taking powerful antibiotics will cure what ails me, and absolutely, definitely, without a doubt will not harm one of the hairs on my chinny chin chin.

I keep my resolve during the subway ride home, the walk to the pharmacy, even throughout the tedious process of dropping off the script. Perhaps the long wait, the rigmarole of setting up an account, entering my insurance info, the helplessness I feel at the out-of-pocket expense are distractions that fortify my resolve. I even hold up while I wait the half-hour for the script to be filled; choosing not to go home, instead I grab a slice, a Coke, and read the *Post* at a nearby pizzeria.

Oh, sure, I'm having difficulty concentrating on yet another Rangers' lackluster performance, swallowing the slice that could use a little more cheese, but I'm holding up. Ask Marlowe, he's sitting at a nearby table, fedora pulled down so low I can't figure out how he can see the daily racing sheet he got at the candy store two doors down.

Unfortunately, when I go to the bathroom at the pizzeria I must piss out the piss and vinegar, because five minutes later when I enter the Duane Reade and head to the rear of the store to pick up my prescription, I begin to unravel.

First, the wobbly, unsteady legs, then the cold ring of throat sweat, and then something new and different and really frightening:

They all have my face! The old, the infirm, the dying—all waiting for me at the pick-up counter. Must be indigestion (happens when I put those red flakes on the pizza), otherwise, why would I be seeing crazy stuff like this? I've been dosed—LSD or some other mind-altering drug. I just saw a story like this on "Law and Order": it's the angry ex, a disgruntled child, a high-school prank, or just a horrifying case of mistaken identity. I expect to see Lennie and Rey approach me as I search for my papaya enzymes, pop a few, then chew them vigorously. No dice—no sharp detectives to save my *tuchis,* although I do visualize giving Briscoe one because he's got some acid. This is good—the papaya should settle my stomach.

But still, Edmond O'Brien is in the house. I'm constantly sweating, already aware of my fast-approaching death, searching frantically for the person responsible for fatally poisoning me. I'm D.O.A.

I must be smiling, because my faces are smiling back at me. I look more closely. Why don't they have my body? I feel tiny sparks of electricity playing leapfrog down my central nervous system. Wait! They're not clones if they don't have my body! What replica only has half your stuff? Is it my imagination, or do I hear popping sounds? I'm short-circuiting and everyone is smiling.

Hail, hail the dope and his doppelgangers. Oooh . . . Oooh . . . Oooh . . . Welcome to the Twilight Zone . . . Oooh . . . Oooh . . . Oooh . . .

I have another question—why do all my faces have tans? I blink once—twice—five times in rapid succession. Someone is offering me a seat—someone without my face. I'm really sweating now. Jesus, am I really D.O.A.? I sit. Nobody seems to be staring at me. That's good. Staring means you're sick, dying, or crazy. Out of the corner of my eye, I sense the brim of a fedora. I turn. In profile, the granite jaw appears to be marked with two razorblade cuts. I can't keep my eyes off the thin crusts of dried blood. How come I didn't see that in the pizzeria? I'm afraid he'll turn and catch me staring, but he's intently looking straight ahead. I follow his gaze. Ex-clones stand shoulder to shoulder, blocking my view of the pick-up counter. I stare at their backs. They begin to meld into one black shape, then the mass lights up like a movie screen.

Wow! A time code appears over my face! The movie begins. Images unravel at the rate of twenty-four frames per second. Scenes long forgotten, perhaps repressed until now—until something snaps in my brain and turns the projector on. *Oooh . . . Oooh . . . Oooh . . .*

Fade-in: I'm in Florida, Hallandale to be exact, and I'm entering a CVS the size of a football field. It will be another four years before I step into a Costco or similar shock-and-maw-dropping humongoloidals, so naturally I'm feeling very virgin vulnerable, though perhaps not as snow white as when, twenty years earlier, I'm overcome with awe upon entering Saint Peter's Basilica. Then again if the roof here is dome-shaped, painted with flying angels holding Viagra, and they erect a giant Revlon Model surmounting the Cathedra Petri sculpted in bronze gilt at the other end of one of the portals (yep, the pharmacy has to have four portals), maybe—maybe then I'll be as rapturously enthralled.

I'm in this CVS to pick up Pop's scripts. I'm clutching a plastic bag containing empty vials and a list of all his meds, plus his Medicare and personal insurance cards. I'm holding it so tightly when I release my grip that there are deep red indentations in my hand. It's the CVS just west of the Hallandale Beach Bridge. Ahh, the HBB . . . Starting with the construction of a second span crossing the

HBB is a scene right out of Escape from New York, *and according to Pop, this traffic nightmare will continue forever as long as the extensive padding makes fat cats fatter.*

Cut.

Now I'm in Pop's indoor garage, surrounded by newly minted convertible Jags, BMWs and Benzes, looking but not touching, feeling my jealousy-level steadily rise until the auto gods mercifully allow me to locate my father's shiny Revlon-red Eldorado, with its cream-colored hardtop. Pimpmobile, Jew canoe, alter-kocker car—whatever scatological hat you want to hang on it, none fit my head; from the moment I get in, I'm embarrassed to all hell to let anyone see me. I want to yell out to all who look my way, "This is my father's Cadillac—I drive a Mercedes Benz!" All right, maybe it's fifteen years old, and the Caddy's brand new—but still it's a Benz and that Benz is I. My personality is molded in Stuttgart. The Mercedes Star is tattooed into my soul, its domination of the land, the sea, and the air is mine by association. I'm Mercedes Young Man—not Cadillac Old Guy.

Fortunately, no one's looking twice in my direction, because the glare from the early-morning sun—in combination with too much caffeine and the natural impatience of a laxative demographic—creates real insanity that threatens to turn the mass of cars heading from A1A to the bridge into a bumper-car attraction. (Did I say it was a scene out of Escape from New York*?)*

Getting out of the garage is no problem, but exiting Pop's condo complex is a little tricky, because there's an electric eye in a post right in front of the guard booth, and unless I get close enough to reach out and touch it when I flash Pop's magnetized parking card in its direction, the eye won't register and the gate remains down until I back up and try again (honking doesn't do it because the booth's unmanned, and if you think about waiting for an attendant, think maybe an hour if you're lucky). However, the really difficult part begins as I make my right out the beachfront condo, because I'm immediately on A1A, and that means I must quickly get to my left so I don't miss the turn lane onto the bridge. This maneuver is a heartbeat away from giving me a stroke, because Floridians don't believe in alternate feed, so merging turns into a giant game of kosher chicken, (assuming these Lilliputians are sitting on pillows and can see over the dashboard, otherwise, it's not kosher at all).

This is the first day I'm driving Pop's car, so I'm amazed to see drivers actually giving me a break when I want to cut in front of them. Could it be that Pop's spanking-new Caddy has some cache amongst the Mercedes and BMW crowd? I'm figuring it's back-in-the-day-nostalgia. These snowbirds are fondly remembering the Fleetwoods, Eldorados, and Coupe de Villes they proudly owned during those halcyon 40s, 50s, and 60s, every year trading them in for a new one—that's what you did back then, when you had the world at your feet and a Caddy in the garage.

Sure, the snarling traffic bothers me, but I love South Florida—always have, ever since that very first time, back in the early 70s, when I came down by train with my ex and our two-year-old son to visit my in-laws. They lived inland, in Fort Lauderdale, but it isn't long before my own family and I go exploring.

Cut.

We're heading east on Commercial all the way over to the fresh ocean breezes, where we pick up A1A going south; a glorious sunlit strip bordered by the Intracoastal on the west and the Atlantic on the east; lush, green palm trees against a blue, sunshine sky painted with a panoply of ever changing fluff-a-duff cloud formations, disappearing like solfège syllables off a musical score into the vanishing ocean's horizon line, behind the gleaming white condos and hotels standing guardian over the coastline beauty.

Eventually, we get down to Hallandale Beach, where, between A1A and the beach, we come face to face with the iconic beach ball-colored water tower soaring into the sky, a South Florida oldies station, blasting tunes of the Fifties and Sixties. Singing along with The Eagles and The Fat Man, invigorating salt ocean breezes blowing through the open windows, I'm young and carefree, and yes—it's a peaceful, easy feeling . . .

Cut.

I'm finally over the bridge onto Hallandale Boulevard; I go (crawl) a couple of blocks, and then make my first right, a jug handle that will get me onto Hallandale in the opposite direction. This is where I must look for the CVS parking lot that should be my second right, making sure not to miss it and be forced to go back over the bridge and retrace my steps—a nightmare that needs no explaining.

Now, when I make my right onto the jug handle, guess where I am? Right next to a mall that conveniently contains Publix and Winn-Dixie, where Pop also has pharmacy accounts. You would think the smart move would be to pull in there, and my father agrees when he gives me these directions and tells me that's what I'll have to do if CVS doesn't have his pills, but—and this is a big, big but—because CVS is cheapest, I'm directed to pass up the first mall and go to CVS first. When I ask why this should matter (I'm under the impression that between Medicare and his own insurance he shouldn't have to pay anything), Pop begins to educate me concerning the intricacies of his medical plans. I cut him off. This is my first close encounter with the Worst Kind, and I have no patience. I can't be bothered with sickness, and I'm certainly not prescient enough to know you mock the thing that will kill you.

Unfortunately, life doesn't let me off so easily. If I'm foolish enough to think living is a series of random acts, that I'm here in Hallandale simply for some Poppy face time and a little R&R on the side, that refusing to see Pop's condition for what it is and how it affects me will just make it disappear—well then, maybe life will just have to get up into my face with a second wake-up call, something a lot less subtle, something between a sharp stick in the eye and a brain embolism. Say, for instance, a nightmarish memory set to come to the surface of my consciousness like the wreckage of a sub after it's split open by a depth charge.

Cut! Roll nightmare!

I'm standing at the empty pick-up counter, removing Pop's vials so I can match them to the ones I'm picking up, an idea I proposed to my father and one he readily appreciated.

I stare at the vials. Deep inside my brain, neurotransmitters are flashing ERIC ROBESPIERRE on an electric billboard lighting up my limbic system, the place where emotions get the best of me—where the chemical equations also spell out the inevitability of bad gene transmission. On the other hand, this is the reptilian part of my brain, and perhaps all it's doing is sensing the close proximity of gators, who, so say the media, love to crawl into CVS parking lots from nearby waterways looking to bite ass and take limbs.

Cut.

I'm sitting outside the CVS, still shaking. The sign on the bench says, **Please give up your seat to the elderly.** *I press my back against the sign so no one can see it. The bag containing Pop's refills plus his old vials sits on my lap. I put on my glasses, check new vials against old. I don't see my name anywhere. What's going on? Why am I still shaking? Why can't I get up, go to the car, drive back to Pop's condo?*

"CAN I HELP YOU?"
Cut.

I'm staring at a pharmacy associate standing under a giant Duane Reade sign. I feel something—*someone*—from behind gripping my shoulder. I half turn— someone old and very wrinkled is smiling at me. I nod at the familiar face of a neighbor from my old building back in the days I lived with my wife in Peter Cooper Village, turn back to the pharmacy associate.

"Uh — uh . . . Robespierre . . . they said it would be ready in half an hour."

My voice seems to be strangely disembodied. The pharmacy associate, a middle-aged African American from America (to distinguish her from native Africans) doesn't react. Am I really speaking?

I glance to my right, at Indian Pharmacy Associate, so I can point to her for verification, but she's not there. Indian Pharmacy Associate's been replaced at the drop-off counter by a drop-dead gorgeous young woman, Indian Pharmacy Associate No. 2. The replacement has a thin streak of red trimming the edges of her short hair. It reminds me of dried blood.

Afro American Woman Pharmacy Associate nods, turns, and looks for the bin associated with my name—only she's looking in the P's. She sifts through the white bags twice without success, turns, and is about to return empty handed

"Robespierre—with an R!" I shout.

She nods weakly, turns back to the bins, this time going for the one marked R.

Robespierre—with an R . . . Who said that? Me . . . I look around. The spell is broken.

I finally take my eyes off the little vial and move it a few inches over on the kitchen counter. My head aches . . . Same shit, different day . . . I need to break the pattern. I open a kitchen cabinet, clear some space, pick up the Cipro and shove it in between the wine glasses and close the door.

Out of sight, out of mind.

ROUND 3

Monday, October 29, 2007, 9:00 a.m. *Throwing a jab...*

I can't point to anything specific—I just wake up this morning and decide to take the Cipro. I read the instructions, or shall I say, *attempt* to read them. First of all, the typeface is so tiny I would need a magnifying lens; second of all, well—as I unfold the sucker, the pages open up like an accordion and I see there are at least six pages, front and back, of tiny type unreadable to my naked eye—and anyone without said magnifying lens. Then there's the ignorance-is-bliss rationale for folding the damn thing up and stuffing it back into the box. I like this choice best.

I make myself a cup of coffee to go with my cold cereal with soy and frozen blueberries, then take the horse-sized pill with some soy that I gulp right out of the container. A man's got to do what a man's got to do.

I think about calling someone, one of my neighbors. Steve would be the best one, just to let him know what I've done, that he should call me every twenty minutes to check up on me; *if I don't answer it's because I got a bad reaction and am lying on the floor in my own pool of whatever it is you lie in when you take this stuff,* and he should come right down (I'll leave the door open) so he can take me to the hospital, by cab—no car, no parking. Which hospital? Beth Israel is closest; Lombardo's at Roosevelt; Dr. Upper East Side, his prescription, what's his hospital? No, Lombardo. Steve will get a cab; I've seen him lift a TV all by himself. No, 911. No, Bellevue. I should call Roosevelt. No, call Lombardo . . . Stop! Stop this thunderous brain chatter. I can feel, *hear* my neurons coming free of their moorings, ricocheting off each other like billiard balls after a break shot in Eight-Ball.

Dr. House in the cranium with a pool cue! Medical migraine! Medical migraine!

This is silly, wimpy, and without any Marlowe-tough redemption. Hundreds of people take this nasty pill, and nothing happens to them—unless, *unless* they're the ones disappearing . . . My God—is this how the aliens kidnap us? Nah, it's got to be the rays the little buggers shoot out of their eyes as they pass us on the street or in a corn field, dissolving us into atoms the mother ship vacuums up. Then, when we're safely locked aboard their spacecraft, they return us to our former selves so they can send us back and spy for them. Gosh, darn—everyone knows that.

Get on with your life, Marlowe-man, check out the Internet Dating Site, see who's been contacting you; even if you don't find love maybe you can use their correspondence for your book.

That's it! Biz as normal—biz as normal . . .

ROUND 4

"I want you to count back from one hundred."

Ninety-nine, ninety-eight, ninety...

I'm out like a light! It's Colonoscopy Time!

Oh, did I forget to tell you? Well, I almost forgot myself. Normally, getting one of these babies is front-page, but unfortunately there's other breaking news these days, so it's on page three or maybe page five, the exact number of years that have gone by since my first one.

I make the appointment when I'm in for my annual Dr. L. checkup, and obviously before I get the results of my PSA—a time of bravery, bluster, and bravado, with the emphasis on bluster and bravado. Let's face it, colonoscopies are no fun, but I must keep a stiff upper lip, pretend it's no big deal. I can still play *let's pretend* because I'm not yet aware of what evil lurks in the heart of my walnut—not even The Shadow does.

This time around the protocol is different. A new, bowel prep (doc's words, not mine) and an anesthesiologist to put me out. Last time the bowel prep is only a few dollars in the store plus the cost of six cans of assorted fruit juices and sodas to wash it down (ugh!). This time there's a prescription, so I know it's going to be pricey.

I may have lost most of my free will, but I do have one or two choices left. I make a command decision. I'm not going back to the Duane Reade on 23rd Street. My Cipro shopping taught me there is some scary Stephen King shit going down in that place. Ghosts, goblins, poltergeists, the devil incarnate—only David Warner would go back for more, and we all remember what happened to him. You think I want to get cut in half by a pane of glass? Oh, what? You think *The Omen* is only a work of fiction? Well, that shows you how much you know!

The Walgreens on First Avenue at 15th Street used to be independently owned and operated and called something else, but remember, this is Chainsaw City: *I came, I saw, I put you out of business.*

Wow, the pharmacy is large, bright, and cheery—best of all, none of the customers wandering around the aisles look like me. I walk up to the counter and immediately a sharply dressed pharmacy aid (name tag says *Simon*) takes my prescription. He wants to know if I'm registered with Walgreens.

"Nope."

"May I see your insurance cards?"

May I? Isn't he the polite one? I'm smiling. This may turn out all right, after all. He doesn't return my smile, and I understand why—he's saving it for the pharmacist, a real stunner of an Indian gal who can't be more than thirty, with full, luscious red lips and tire-size gold hoop earrings, and who speaks so softly I'm wondering if Simon can hear her. Next thing I know, I'm applying henna to her naked body, something I've become expert in after watching *Monsoon Wedding* more times than I care to admit. I like this pharmacy.

"I want you to count back from one hundred."

Ninety-nine, ninety-eight, ninety . . .

I blink a few times, letting the bright light slowly make its way into my brain. It's alive! It's alive! Colin Clive is in the house! Okay, there's no lab, I'm no resurrected Frankenstein, but nevertheless, it is a eureka moment. Gene and Marty are suddenly in the house: "*Fronkensteen.*" "*You're putting me on.*"

Waking up is fun to do—remember the alternative.

ROUND 5

MY brainstorm of an idea is to have breakfast, then hang around the house until I muster up enough courage to go uptown and take my *après*-Cipro PSA test. But somewhere between the making of the coffee and the actual drinking of my morning brew, a little warning light flashes in my brain, or maybe it's a bell going *ring-ring* or a voice (*come on, we all hear them*), urging me to call Dr. Upper East Side's office just to make sure there won't be any problems. Sure, Dr. Upper East Side said I didn't need an appointment, and sure, all I have to do is tell the front desk, but you have to be a total moron to dismiss the brain-chattering cautions (I've learned the hard way), and sure enough, when I follow my instincts, the receptionist says any time during office hours, except between twelve and one, when the nurses take their lunch.

As I head up to the doctor's office, I tell myself that making the call and getting the correct info is a good omen. Now, most of you probably don't see it that way. A smart move, a cautionary one, we can all agree upon, but a good omen? Boy, that's a stretch. No, on second thought it's too much of a stretch to be even considered a smart move. Under ordinary circumstances, I'd agree with you. On the other hand, there are times I'm holding onto sanity by a thread and I'll do anything to keep my grip.

This good-omen thing is giving me such positive feelings that I'm not even thinking about body-snatching. I mean it. Right next to me, also walking toward the Lexington Avenue subway, is another group of robust, college guys—perfect targets for a takeover, but it never crosses my mind. Instead, I'm walking step by step with them, as if I'm one of their group, healthy and carefree. This is great!

The waiting room is jammed. Does every man over the age of forty have bad walnuts? It looks like it.

"Hi, I'm Eric Robespierre, and I'm a patient of Dr. Upper East Side's. I'm here for a follow-up PSA test."

I've been practicing the spiel since I got off the subway. I pause at a red light. It's a beautiful day on the Upper East Side, with the six-figure cars depositing seven-figure women in front of eight-figure town houses. The fancy-dancy store windows glisten with products the ordinary cannot afford, and which the extraordinary collect like lint in a public dryer. I once saw Robert Duvall walking these very streets. I followed him at a distance, and when he got to 72nd and Madison, I fully expected him to whirl around in front of the Ralph Lauren Store and intone: "I love the smell of money on the Upper East Side—it smells like victory!"

The light turns green. I cross Mad Ave. My head is down and I'm once more muttering: "Hi, I'm Eric Robespierre, and I'm a patient of Dr. Upper East Side's. I'm here for a follow-up PSA test." Thank God the beautiful people never look at me.

Once I arrive, I finally get to say my spiel (as rehearsed) when I get the attention of a nurse who normally wouldn't give me the time of day (remember the sign-in instructions), but I'm lucky enough to catch her just after she's dressed down a poor guy who didn't read the sign—in the moment when she looks straight at me, as if wanting me to acknowledge her raw power. Instead, I catch her off-guard.

"I'm Eric Robespierre, and I'm a patient of Dr. Upper East Side's. I'm here for a follow-up PSA test."

I know she wants to take my head off, but she can't. However, what she *can* do is get even by giving me instructions at a decibel level inaudible to the human ear. I can either pretend I heard her and go into the back and take my chances, or ask her to repeat herself. This little routine obviously gives her her jollies; the smirk on her face gives it away. Then she turns away and picks up a ringing phone. I'm not going to give the b-i-t-c-h the satisfaction. I turn to the left, head into the warren-like maze, and immediately see a woman in white.

"I'm Eric Robespierre, and I'm a patient of Dr. Upper East Side's. I'm here for a follow-up PSA test."

How lucky, this is the very person who does the bloodletting. No, she isn't covered in the red stuff, has no leeches attached to her smock, and isn't long in the fang—she's just your good old-fashioned nurse with a friendly smile and a lolli tucked in her breast pocket. Okay, I'm lying about the lolli, but guess what, there *is* a jar of them in the tiny bloodletting room. At first I don't see them. I'm too busy removing my coat while out of the corner of my eye I watch her prepare the syringe. I'm really nervous now. I begin nonstop talking. She's sniffling. I talk about winter colds and how hard it must be to work when you're sick. Joan, that's her name, has an accent (my guess: second-generation Irish outta Queens), and it doesn't take her long to complain about her job, her cold, and how both are interrupting the holiday shopping season.

She checks out my right arm, and before I can say, "rolling veins," shakes her head.

"Left arm, please."

"You got it."

I look away (who wants to see your blood streaming out of your body?), and that's when I spot the lollies. My first thought is they're for the kids, so maybe I shouldn't ask for one. Suddenly the song by the Chordettes fills my head, and I can't stop singing it.

> *"Lollipop, Lollipop, oh lolli-lolli-lolli*
> *Lollipop, Lollipop, oh lolli-lolli-lolli*
> *Lollipop, Lollipop, oh lolli-lolli-lolli*
> *Lollipop*
> *Come and be my Lollipop, tell you why*
> *Kisses sweeter than an apple pie*
> *And when she does her shakin' rockin' dance*
> *Man, I haven't got a chance*
> *I call her Lollipop, Lollipop, oh lolli-lolli-lolli*
> *Lollipop, Lollipop, oh lolli-lolli-lolli*
> *Lollipop, Lollipop, oh lolli-lolli-lolli*
> *Lollipop"*

For the life of me I can't remember any more. All I can hear are the Chordettes, clapping away as they repeat the refrain. Then my mind goes to when I was a teenager and to my father—who worked for my mother's father, who owned Madame Kuglers, a French hand-laundry store on the north side of West 74th Street, one hundred feet west of Columbus Avenue as the city pigeon flies. Back in the day (before dry-cleaning stores) "hand-laundry stores" catered to the very rich, and among his famous clients was Archie Blyer, the owner of Cadence Records. Mr. Blyer, who was also married to one of the Chordettes, was gracious enough to give my father complimentary 45s of his company's latest releases—which leads me down the next neuron trail to The Everly Brothers, a country-rock influenced duo whose first song, "Bye Bye Love," I must have played nonstop from the time I got home until bedtime, on a cheap portable record player that today probably sounds so tinny as to be unbearable to listen to. I set the record player up in the middle of my floor and I sprawled out next to it. I used to get the Everly Brothers records before they hit the airwaves, and that made me a big cheese at school. Besides the Chordettes and the Everly Brothers, there was Johnny Tillotson and Link Wray and his Ray Men.

Nurse Bloodletting notices I'm looking at the lollipops and offers me one. I'm not making a move until she removes the needle and finishes her job. I'm also not going to look in that direction until I'm absolutely positive my blood doesn't runneth over anymore.

"Hold, please."

I look over and she's pressing down on a nice size piece of cotton. I do as she orders. Painless.

"You're good," I tell her.

"Don't think that'll get you two lollipops."

"Oh, please? I'm schizophrenic."

She laughs, and applies a small band-aid to the puncture site.

"So when can I call for the results? Or will Dr. Upper East Side call me?"

"Two weeks to ten days, but don't quote me." She lowers her voice to a conspiratorial whisper. "When he gets the results, he forwards it and his own instructions to a typing service, who writes it all up, sends it back to him, and then he signs it and mails it out to you."

Now I remember. This is what the receptionist told me, but I thought that was how he delivered routine news, not something like results that might lead to a biopsy.

My face must be a mess of frowns. Ms. Bloodletting understands my disappointment and hands me the jar of lollies. I pick two yellows.

"I know what Dr. Upper East Side does may not suit you, but that's how he operates." She smiles, lays a comforting hand on mine.

Like it or lump it. Right? Wrong! I pull on my sweater and then put on my coat. I may be too downtrodden to man the barricades, but there are other ways to show I'm mad as hell and won't take it anymore. The warrior is trained to use what's at hand when engaging in hand-to-hand combat. I remove the covering of a lolli—not so easy because there's a tiny sliver stuck to the surface, and if I'm not careful, I'll end up dislodging it with my saliva and swallowing it. We've all been down that slippery path, right? I gently tug on either side of the offending portion until it comes loose. I examine my weapon: locked, loaded, and lick perfect. I begin to suck. It's a violent, slurpy suck.

Suck on this, Dr. Upper East Side!

ROUND 6

Wednesday, November 29, 2007, 2:00 p.m. *One to the stomach . . .*

Dear Mr. Robespierre:

Your current prostatic-specific antigen, obtained when you had taken a two-week course of the antibiotic Cipro, did not show a favorable downward trend; indeed, your current PSA actually increased slightly to the value of 4.67 ng/ml.

Your PSA value in October of this year has been 3.91 ng/ml; thus, rather than going down with your taking antibiotics for two weeks, your PSA actually increased.

Although you continue to have an excellent ratio of free to total PSA—namely, 28%—I am somewhat concerned about your upward PSA trend.

What I would want you to do is to drop by our office again at the end of December to have another PSA value drawn. Should your PSA numbers continue to increase, then a biopsy of your prostate would be absolutely mandatory.

With warm personal regards,

Sincerely yours,

Dr. Upper East Side

I'm standing in my lobby, in front of my open mailbox. I have to take out my glasses to read the letter. Usually I'll open up the correspondence and try it *sans* peepers. This never works, but I'm vain (yes, this song is about me), and I continue to play this silly game—until now. Suddenly, I'm growing smarts. Suddenly, I'm acting in a responsible manner. I'm scared—plain and simple.

I read the letter twice. I'd like to read it a few more times so I don't just get every fourth word, but there's a limit to the time I can stand in front of the lobby mailboxes when a total collapse of the body could put me on the floor at any moment. Messy. And what about my nosey neighbors? What would they say, and say and say . . . ? There's more mail, but I'm not interested, especially in the bills I fantasize tearing up and dumping in the trash. Dead-man's revenge!

I shove the bills back into the mail slot, close it up, and carefully put my keys in my left jean pocket. I'm well aware that in times I'm most stressed, I'm sure to become distracted, and losing my keys is a distinct possibility. Losing my wallet is another real concern, so I tell myself I have to pay strict attention when I take it out. I pat my right jean pocket and feel the comforting bulge. I have to pay strict attention.

"Shit, shit, and double shit!"

I look around. Thank God no one is in the lobby.

I have two library books in my hand and it was my intention to return them. Now I'm not sure what to do. I could go back upstairs, curl into a ball and sleep. Sleep is my first line of defense, my best psychic hiding place. I still have the letter in my hand. I put it back into its envelope, fold it, and stick it right down next to my wallet. Not a good idea. I take the letter and wallet out, then slide letter into wallet. It's not a good fit, but at least I'm sure I won't lose the letter. That would be terrible. I don't want anyone to know my business.

"With warm personal regard . . ." What an odd way of signing someone's death sentence. Okay, I'm exaggerating, but this valediction is a little too kissy-kissy for my taste, unless you translate kissy-kissy to kiss-off—or kiss of death. Okay, I'm exaggerating again! I can't catch a break, even when I'm arguing with myself.

Of course, I knew Dr. Upper East Side's letter was coming. I had been living in fear of its arrival for nearly a week now, but each day it hadn't come gave me another twenty-four-hour chunk of peace. Well, not really—each day that passed fueled my growing pessimism. I think about seeing a shrink. I try to bury myself in my writing and that's the only thing that works—sometimes. *Paul Atreides is in the house.*

"I must not fear. Fear is the mind-killer. Fear is the little death that brings total obliteration. I will face my fear. I will permit it to pass over me and through me. And when it has gone past I will turn the inner eye to see its path. Where the fear has gone there will be nothing. Only I will remain. Fear is the mind-killer. It's only an infection."

I have it written on the back of Dr. Upper East Side's card, but I don't have to take the card out—I have Herbert's words memorized to a T.

It's Dr. Upper East Side in the head with a gom jabbar. Dune migraine! Dune migraine!

"With warm personal regards . . . " Now what? One step closer to the biopsy—that's what. My worst fears realized—that's what. My pessimism validated—that's what. Sure, it could still be an infection. The letter says wait, get tested again and then see, doesn't it? *Sure. And if pigs could fly they would be eagles. Bullshit. You want to go through another month of this agony? Hold it, Masked Man!* I have an idea! Maybe I should just go in and have the damn thing done tomorrow? *How's that for an idea? Huh? Huh? Huh?*

That's a real stupid idea. Think what the letter says. The letter says you'll need a biopsy. Does not! *Does so!*

I find myself walking toward the Stuyvesant Town Oval. If the fountain in the Oval is working, maybe I'll just jump in?

"I must not fear. Fear is the mind-killer . . ." Dune *Migraine!* Dune *Migraine!*

I sleepwalk through the remainder of the day, but despite my somnambulistic state I manage not to lose my keys or my wallet. I don't faint away on the sidewalk. I don't walk into traffic and get whacked by a bus. I don't go to a local bar and get pissed. I don't go home and finish off the half-bottle of Merlot and then collapse in a pool of my own vomit. I don't call my kids or my friends and cry like a baby. Why dull the pain or share it when I can totally brutalize myself by imagining the biopsy in all its gory details? . . . . Grabbing onto the sides of the examining table, teeth grinding, butt cheeks tightening, stabbing pain, screaming out in agony; naturally, I'm living this in living color *mit* Dolby. Maybe in space no one can hear you scream, but when that freaky fangy thing comes out of your ass in the urologist's office, you can bet even Sigourney Weaver would yell her head off.

One thing about obsessing about biopsies: you don't have time to think about bad walnuts.

ROUND 7

Tuesday, December 24, 2007, 1:00 p.m. *Take my blood, please . . .*

I'M so jealous of all these smiley faces: on the street, in restaurants, bodegas, even in the subways, smiley faces—smiley faces everywhere. Not me. I can't remember the last time I smiled, really smiled, a full mind-and-body smile, the kind you have when you're happy and not worried about a goddamn thing.

I've seen pictures of me like that. There's one on a tricycle, dressed in checked jacket with a mouton collar. I must be five or six, and I'm grinning from ear to ear as I tool around 74th and Columbus Avenue on a blustery, wintry morning. There's a photo of me with my high school pals, in Long Beach, Long Island, at the water's edge, wearing retro twenties swimsuits that come down to the knees, something very much in fashion for maybe a year. What about the ones when I'm holding one of my children, or maybe posing with both in the playground at Peter Cooper Village? I'm smiling pretty good in those photos. My wedding photo—no, I think I look a little serious in that one, but there's a bunch from our honeymoon, and I'm smiling ear to ear in those shots.

There's holiday music everywhere, even the car-horn blowing sounds festive. And the kids—every kid you see is laughing and jumping around like they've got ants in their pants. How can you not smile when you see kids like that? *Easy, thy names are jealously and self-pity. You even begin to hate happy people. How can they be so cheery when you might have bad walnuts? How selfish and uncaring of them. Do I have to be nailed to a cross to get some sympathy, people?*

What's the expression—misery loves company? Good luck finding some during the holidays. Maybe that's why so many unhappy people commit suicide now. If they could just hold out until a week or two—until after the holidays, when the euphoria and the booze bliss has worn off and people slide back into their sinkholes—then, then see how many smiling faces you run into on the subway.

Wait a minute, Masked Man, there's hope—misery is just around the corner.

I enter Dr. Upper East Side's office. The place is packed with grump-a-dumps like me. Nobody's smiling here—you betcha, by gum, by golly. Okay, they may not be thinking about me, but the important thing is they're as frightened and fucked up as yours truly— and you know what? That's good enough for me. Misery is not picky about the company it seeks.

I walk right up to the desk and smile. It's a perverse, wicked smile. Immediately, I get attention. All eyes look up, stare at me. There is something about wickedness that demands attention.

"I'm Eric Robespierre, I'm a patient of Dr. Upper East Side's and I'm here to get my PSA checked."

ROUND 8

Dear Mr. Robespierre:

Your current prostatic-specific antigen, obtained on December 24, 2007, has been reported to be 6.4 ng/ml.

This PSA reading is a further elevation as compared to the value that has been recorded in October of this past year (3.91 ng/ml).

Although you continue to have a favorable ratio of free to total PSA (39%), unfortunately this current PSA value demands a biopsy of your prostate gland.

A prostate biopsy is an office procedure, which is done with the help of local anesthesia to reduce the discomfort caused by the needle passing into the prostate gland.

In preparation for a biopsy, you must not take any medications which interfere with blood clotting, especially aspirin. If you are taking aspirin, you should stop taking the medication now and wait two weeks before undergoing a prostate biopsy.

Also in preparation for a prostate biopsy, you should be taking an antibiotic the day before, the day of the biopsy, and a few days after the biopsy. The antibiotic is Levaquin (500 mg daily) and I have enclosed a prescription for this antibiotic to be taken over these few days.

With warm personal regards,

Sincerely yours,

Dr. Upper East Side

I'm back in my apartment, lying down on my bed, my shoes and overcoat still on. I'm not moving an inch. The bad news letter lies on my stomach. The lights are off, but there's plenty of sunlight coming from the windows. This is my refuge. This is where I go to escape.

Not today.

I told you—I knew it—bad fucking walnuts—you have cancer—you're going to have a biopsy—I told you so—it's going to hurt like hell—you have cancer— like your father—I told you so.

Dr. World of Hurt in my cranium with a psyche scythe. Mind-psych migraine! Mind-psych migraine!

NO, NO, NO!

"I must not fear. Fear is the mind-killer. Fear is the little death that brings total obliteration. I will face my fear. I will permit it to pass over me and through me. And when it has gone past I will turn the inner eye to see its path. Where the fear has gone there will be nothing. Only I will remain. Fear is the mind-killer. It's only an infection."

Dune migraine! Dune migraine!

Marlowe sits down on the other side of the bed, throws his feet up, and lays his head back on the pillow. I have a king-size bed, but I can feel the weight shift. I don't have to open my eyes to know what's going on.

"You okay, pally? You're not gonna throw a joe?"

"I'm just thinking."

"Yeah?"

"Yeah . . . "

"If you're gonna pass out you might as well do it on the bed."

"I'm not going to pass out. I'm just thinking."

"You said that. What are you thinking, pally?"

"I'm not going back to Dr. Upper East Side."

"You're not shining me on?"

"I've got to find another urologist, one with a better bad-news manner—one that's going to put me out with drugs."

"You're not gonna take a bounce, are you?"

"I'm not having a biopsy unless I'm out cold."

"Sounds reasonable, pally."

"I'm going to make some calls."

"You gonna drink?"

"Maybe some coffee."

"Stay off the juice."

"You don't need to tell me.

"It's gonna be all right, you know. Don't worry."

"Yeah?"

"Yeah."

Streams of sunlight bathe Marlowe's shiny, black brogues, turning them into reflecting pool of gleaming leather. Tiny sparkles shoot up into the air. I try to count the dust particles that hang in the air above me. His shoes—he's got to get them shined professionally.

"You know, it's bad luck to put shoes on the bed."

"They got feet in them, pally."

"Oh, so now you know all about Jewish superstitions?" I close my eyes.

I feel the weight shift. He's getting off the bed. I open my eyes. His grey fedora is pulled down so low I can't figure how he sees anything.

"Just don't do a gas run—you don't want to blow the house down."

"Lemme have your gun, then."

He stops at the doorway. "Suppose you miss, pally. Send one through the wall and kill that nice social-worker lady next door."

"You think?"

 He doesn't answer. He just leaves.

I get out of bed, go into every room, pull up the shades and open up the windows; nothing bad hides in the light. I'm feeling better.

Call Ira. I find his work number, punch it in, talking out loud until my voice is frog-free: "Fear is the mind-killer, fear is the mind-killer—you give us twenty-two minutes we'll give you the world."

The receptionist answers on the first ring and puts me through right away. Ira tells me he's heading out for a meeting. I hear the anxiety in his voice, so I try to be brief. I tell him about the letter. He mellows out, but I figure I have two minutes at best.

"I'm not crazy about my urologist, so could I have the name of your guy, phone number, address?"

"Dr. Berman, on 10th or 11th Street—call Sharon if you can't find the number in the phone book. How are you feeling?"

"Okay."

"It's probably nothing. It doesn't have to be cancer."

"I know."

"You'll have to have the biopsy."

"Look, how painful are these things?"

"It was over a year ago." He's trying to avoid telling me the truth. "It wasn't bad," he says finally.

"Yeah?"

"Uh-huh."

"Did he put you out?"

"No."

"No?"

"How long did it take?"

"I don't remember. He did it right in his office."

"He did?"

"Yep. Ask Sharon, she was in the waiting room."

"So, it really wasn't so bad?"

I hear voices in the background pressuring Ira to hang up. "I know you have to go. Thanks—I feel a lot better."

"Call Sharon., I think she's home now. Call me later if you want—I get home around six."

"I will."

I decide to call Ellyn instead of Sharon. I'm trying to stay calm, but it's not easy. I have dry mouth, and the froggies are back.

"Hello, this is Eric Robespierre. Three score and six years into my life, my forefathers shoved a tube up my you-know-what, and I haven't been able to sit down since."

My words aren't exactly rolling off my tongue. It's more like they're traveling through a mouthful of cotton candy. I have in my head the image of bats, imprinted with letters of the alphabet, hanging upside down, stuck to the roof of the bat cave, then one by one they start to fall off. I find myself working my jaw to keep it from closing. I think about looking up the symptoms for lockjaw.

I get Ellyn's voice mail and manage to leave a relatively coherent message. Stay on task: Check. Get info on Dr. Berman: Check. What else? Find out the name of the doctor that treated Mayor Giuliani for his prostate? Check. Ask if he's the same one DeNiro goes to: Check. Ask if he puts you out: Double check.

I turn on my computer. While it's booting up, I go into the kitchen and make some coffee. Out my kitchen window I can see a seaplane coming in from the south and heading upriver for a landing. I wave at the gleaming shape as it zips by. I see the bottle of red on the counter. I'm thinking, *In vino veritas. Truth—I don't need no stinkin' truth!*

I discover Bobby's been treated at Sloan-Kettering Memorial Hospital, but there's no reference to his doctor or to how his case is handled. Rudy's even more difficult—I can't find doctor or hospital, but I do sniff out that Mayor G.

chose hormone treatment, followed by radiation and then seed implantation. My research leads me to articles about the robotic surgery that doctors at Sloan-Kettering recently perfected, which is reputed to be less invasive and apparently lessens some of the serious side effects. But no matter how favorable this sounds, I have already decided against surgery for a few reasons: The side effects are more serious when they cut, especially the chance of impotency and incontinence. Then there is the pain issue; I hear that's a bitch. Hormone treatments, radiation treatments, and seed implantation aren't without their own nasty side effects, either, however, there's no doubt in my mind that they're the lesser of the two evils. The clincher for me is there doesn't seem to be a difference in the survival rate between the two choices, as confirmed by three different research articles, all published within the last six months.

Dr. Howard I. Scher's name keeps popping up in various articles. I Google him and discover he is Chief of the Genitourinary Oncology Service at the Memorial Sloan-Kettering Cancer Center in New York. For the heck of it, I call Sloan-Kettering and get hit with a recorded voice that provides me with a staggering menu of choices; however, these people know that they're dealing with frightened crazies like me, so they make sure Recorded Voice is heaven-sent. I feel my eyelids getting heavier and heavier.

"For Urology, hit seven."

That's it!

I'm connected almost immediately, and get another angelic voice—this one live. I tell my newest angel my story, and she's on top of it right way.

"Dr. Scher is an oncologist. I need to get you one of the urologists for the biopsy. There is Dr. A and Dr. B. Would you like me to connect you with one?"

I'm caught off guard and have to regroup. I ask her to spell the doctors' names and to give me their extensions.

"Oh, by the way, do you know if either of these doctors puts you out for the biopsy?"

"No, but I'm sure their office will know. Would you like me to connect you?"

"Uhh, sure . . . "

Amazing, I'm put right through. Now, if they only put me out.

"I need a biopsy of my prostate. I'd like to be totally sedated during the procedure."

His Wussiet has spoken, but like Rodney, I get no respect—even though I substitute "totally sedated" for "put out." Instead she wants to know if I'm already a patient of Doctors A or B.

"No, I'm not a patient."

"Let's see, for Doctor A I can fit you in a week from this Thursday, at 12:00 p.m., and for Doctor B, I can get you in—ha, also that same day, but at 4:00 p.m."

No more pussyfooting for this pussy.

"I'd like to be put out."

"I'm sorry, but the procedure is so short and really not very painful, so the doctors don't use anything but a local."

"Oh . . . " I'm totally bummed. I thought I could find someone who could help me out here, but now that looks impossible. "Okay, thank you. You've been very kind. I'll get back to you . . ." (pause/click as I hang up) "when I grow a set."

Round 9

STRANGE things are happening. This is the first time I'm going to a doctor whose office isn't located on the Upper East Side—where all the best hospitals are found—but rather to one in the West Village, where one block north the best drag-queen clothier is located.

Of course, this is not strange, just plain wrong-headed of me to think so, and I'm ashamed of my close-minded, out-of-date viewpoint. When I look up Dr. Berman/Saint Vincent's Comprehensive Cancer Center, I discover both make numerous best-doctor/hospital lists so I'm overjoyed and incredibly relieved to get an appointment so quickly. Naturally, I name drop, mentioning Ira and a Dr. Brown (Ellyn's contact, and a former associated of Dr. Berman's) any chance I get. I intend to "your friend is my friend" and brown nose my way into their hearts.

As soon as I make the appointment with Dr. Berman, I feel a great sense of relief and experience a sense of calmness, something I never had when I saw Dr. Upper East Side, and as I turn onto 9th Street, the calmness amazingly is still with me. I realize I'm one who requires order and balance. My Libra nature demands it, and obviously this need takes precedence over my neurotic fear of pain—at least for this moment.

I think I know the building I'm headed for. It's a white residential complex, maybe fourteen floors in height, and takes up almost the entire south side of the block between Broadway and University Place. It's also just a block away from the antique dealer I worked for a few years back, and those fond memories are still very fresh in my head, and for a silly second I consider popping in and unburdening myself to the owner who, I haven't seen since I left.

Instead, I immediately cross over to the south side of the street and head west in the direction of the huge white complex, but when I check the number on the awning I'm dismayed. This isn't the place. I'm completely fooled. How could I be so wrong?

I check the address the receptionist gave me over the phone, and I realize it's an even number and has to be on the other side of the street. I wait for the traffic to stop, jaywalk between the tight rows of cars and trucks to the other side, and head back up toward Broadway. It's got to be the big red brick at the corner, so I naturally pass the side door with the white frame molding without checking the address and approach the main entrance, only to be turned around by a spiffy doorman attired in enough gold braid to make the Joint Chiefs envious.

"It's the little white door," he says, pointing as his friendly smile wrinkles his face up to his eyebrows. "Don't feel bad, everyone makes the same mistake."

Easy for you to say, *Mon General!*

So much for being calm. I'm obviously not thinking straight. I dutifully follow instructions, reach the right address, press the correct series of intercom buttons, and finally reach my destination. The office waiting room is narrow and filled with dour-looking men of all ages. When will I stop being surprised by this image, which reminds me of those beaten-down souls waiting on depression-era bread lines?

I take a deep breath. I know Marlowe is right with me. I walk straight up to the reception area. The clock on the wall says 5:45 p.m.; I'm fifteen minutes early. Two young women are sitting there, one in street clothes, the other an angelic blonde, lovely in pale blue scrubs; both are all smiles when I introduce myself. Guess what else—there aren't any foreboding sign-in signs either. *Gee, Masked Man, we're not on the Upper East Side anymore!*

I know the drill. I sign in, get the necessary forms, fill them out, hand over my insurance cards, and wait. I look around. No eye contact here, either, so I'm left to make up my own scenarios. These are downtown people, more casual in dress and demeanor, and younger than uptown. Grim faces, yes, but less demonstrable angst; are they able to deal with stuff better, or is their stuff less threatening? There's a rack of magazines, some pleasant-looking watercolors on the walls— nothing special in the way of interior design, but certainly not as drab as the last office. The waiting area is also significantly smaller than its uptown counterpart. I think I saw three names under the intercom here, while there had to be three to the power of infinity uptown.

Speaking of uptown, I have all of Dr. Upper East Side's correspondence, and I intend to give the letters to Dr. Berman so he can fully evaluate my condition. They're in my cargo bag and there they stay—no sense in stirring up the anxiety pot.

I have my regular gear in there, too: mystery book, iPod, and this time two issues of *The New Yorker* . . . only I'm not in the mood for any of it yet. I glance around the room. There are three rows of four seats facing the office area. There isn't room at the ends, and I didn't feel like squeezing by anyone, so I take a seat in one of the vacant chairs along the opposite wall. I can see why these seats are unoccupied. You look up and you're staring at a line of grim profiles, faces that at any moment can turn and give you the *Malocchio*. There's a third set of chairs, but they're directly facing the three rows; this is a choice that is no choice, unless you're able to keep your head down and avoid any evil eye contact, something this Nosey Parker can't do.

When I fill out the forms, they no longer seem daunting or frightening, nor are they an object of ridicule. I fill them out carefully, but mechanically, as if on autopilot. It's almost as if it's not me who scratches out the answers. It's certainly not me who sits serenely in this chair, already resigned to the biopsy—already convinced that I have cancer eating away at my walnut, the image of which is now glued somewhere deep in my amygdala. Before I heard the prostate referred to as walnut in shape and size, this tiny gland was impossible to visualize in my mind's eye, but now, when I think of cancer working its way through my prostate, I imagine a walnut, the shell cracking, then the nutty layers turning black and falling out through the breach.

I wait for almost half an hour in a semi-catatonic state, my brain switching between walnuts and the choreographed flow of sober-looking men of all ages, races, and creeds going in and out of examining rooms, bathrooms, and private offices. As patients leave, new bodies replace them in an elegantly timed exchange, all orchestrated by Dr. Berman's efficient staff. I admire their expertise and wonder if they should be running the DOT. The thought of receptionists operating our traffic system makes me giggle. I think I'm losing it.

"Mr. Rass-berry?"

Some things never change. I stand and instinctually raise my hand and weakly smile at a dark-haired woman in pale-blue scrubs. She is already turning to lead me toward one of the examination rooms. She's holding a manila file folder against her ample chest.

"Robespierre . . . I know it's a tough one,"

It's the sight of big breasts, otherwise why would I lose control and stupidly try to correct someone with access to needles.

She half-turns and faces me. I'm fucked.

"Robespierre . . . " She smiles.

I let out a lungful of air. "Perfect."

"Robespierre," she says again.

"You got it—now you can use my credit card."

We both laugh and I'm back to breathing normally.

She studies my chart, checking to make sure she has it right, then leads me into one of the exam rooms. I enter a narrow corridor. Facing me is a row of other examination rooms. I'm suddenly not feeling funny anymore. Out of the corner of my right eye I see the blur of a grey fedora.

"Lose the grip, pally." Do I see him smiling at me? "For there is nothing either good or bad, but thinking makes it so."

Is he kidding? Then he's gone, but his words hang out there in the empty hallway like skywriting on a cloudless day. I like him better when he's not playing the bard. I look around for clues that indicate this room is special, signs that provide a heads-up on the kind of exam I can anticipate, but I'm not really sure what I'm looking for.

"Please take everything off, down to your shorts and t-shirt. You can keep your socks on."

Good news. God knows what killer bacteria lives on the white linoleum.

"Dr. Berman will be with you shortly." She smiles, then slides my chart down into a plastic holder fastened to the outside of the door, and closes it.

I put my large, grey Hugo Boss overcoat on the back of an uncomfortably smallish metal chair that sits under a bare window looking out into a darkened courtyard; so much for atmosphere. *It's just you and me, Hugo.* I slowly remove my clothes and carefully lay them over my coat: first my fleece sweater, then my turtleneck, then my pants, all neatly folded as if I'm laying out my clothes for an event—my funeral? Last but not least, I sit, remove my shoes, and shove them under the chair. I retrieve Dr. Upper East Side's letters from the cargo bag and clutch them in my cold hands.

I can wait for Dr. Berman standing up, sitting on the examining table (I'm certainly not relaxed enough to recline), or I can chose the little metal chair. I think I will sit on the chair, even though I'll have to lean against all my clothes. The metal feels cold. This isn't going to work. I open my cargo bag again and get my glasses and Ian Rankin book. I'm going to have to sit on the examining table.

I hoist myself up, put on my glasses, and open the book. I carefully place Dr.

Upper East Side's correspondence next to me on the table. I dangle my feet and think of Tom Sawyer sitting on the edge of the dock, fishing. All I need is a pole and a straw hat.

Not quite, Masked Man . . .

I open Mr. Rankin to where my bookmark shows I left off, and stare at the first line of text. I don't know why I think I can concentrate. I'm cold and on the verge of shivering. I'm wondering if anyone has written a self-help book on how to psychologically overcome the anxiety that's steadily building inside me: *Zen and The Art of Doctors' Waiting Rooms* would be a good one. *Chillin' While Illin': How To Avoid Exam-Room Hysteria* is another. Maybe I should think about writing one?

Obviously, the medical equipment is something you must avoid looking at, because that only leads to terrifying torture-chamber imagery, and with all the spy books, movies, and TV series I have been addicted to over my adult lifetime—well, you get the point. I'll tell you this, if Dr. Berman looks like Kiefer Sutherland, it's not going to take me twenty-four hours to have a heart attack.

The walls are paper-thin, and every time I hear voices in the hallway I stiffen in anticipation. I hop off the table. The door remains closed. False alarm. There are the obligatory cabinets stocked with drugs, bandages, and syringes of all sizes—necessary, comforting items if you only associate them with healing and don't think about the other stuff, like writhing in pain as your life's blood drains out your body. The life-size diagrams of the human body are always a treat. This one is particularly innovative, because the cranium reminds me of the creature from *Alien*. I stare at the prostate gland and see a cracked walnut stuck to the illustration. Two blinks and it's gone.

Too much information makes a person nuts (no pun intended).

I try to remember if Dr. Upper East Side has any similar illustrations. He most likely did, just like every dentist has at least one illustration of a set of teeth, urologists have their prostate, penis, et al. I wonder if the docs get them free, courtesy of a drug company? There's something at the bottom of this illustration, but I can't make it out. I know if I were doing the marketing for, say, the lab that produces Viagra, I'd put their name on every illustration. Would I also add a stiff penis? The thought makes me smile.

I close my eyes, but for the life of me, I don't remember much about Dr.

Upper East Side's examining room, probably because I was busy freaking about his German accent, imagining all sorts of crazy things the guy did during the war. I grimace. My God, did I actually think of calling him Mein Führer? Why am I so mean? Dr. Upper East Side is probably the nicest man alive and despises the evil Nazis as much as anyone. Too much Jewish Defense Mechanism in me. Thank God I didn't totally lose it and begin hearing "Springtime For Hitler and Germany" in my head, or even worse, go totally berserk and start singing and dancing around his treatment room.

I smile, imagining that crazy scene, wondering how Dr. Upper East Side would react to such a nut job. Absentmindedly, I begin humming a few bars as I carelessly gaze around the room. My eyes finally stop at a particularly creepy piece of machinery sitting against the wall under the *Alien* illustration. Suddenly, a new song pops into my head and out of my lips.

"The Inquisition (Let's Begin)
The Inquisition (Look out sin)
We have a mission
To convert the Jews (Jew Jew Jew Jew Jew Jew Jew)
We're gonna teach them (Wrong from right)
We're gonna help them (See the light)
And make an offer that they can't refuse. (That the Jews just can't refuse)
Confess, don't be boring
Say yes, don't be dull."

More voices outside. I stop singing (it was more of a low murmur than an Ethel Merman belter). I hop back up on the table. *Wipe that grin off your face and take a few deep breaths. Get yourself together.*

The door opens. Roy Scheider staring into the bathroom mirror replaces images of Mr. Mel Brooks. *Goodbye, Torquemada—hello, Bob Fosse.*

Showtime for Marlowe!

Surprise, surprise, he's younger and more handsomely debonair than I expect. I hope my expression isn't taken as a show of disapproval. *Shit, shit, triple-shit!* Serves me right if I screw the pooch here with another faulty stereotypical belief I'm so good at producing. Paraphrasing Peter: *This is the quicksand upon which I build my psyche; no wonder it's so fragile.*

"Hi, I'm Eric Robespierre." I smile. Extend my hand.

Dr. Berman stares at my file. He looks up, nods, and shakes my hand firmly. But there is no fellowship of the ring here. Only one way to save the situation . . .

"Dr. Brown says hello. He's in Florida." My words stumble out in two incomplete thoughts, but the message gets through.

Dr. Berman looks up, smiles.

Got ya!

"You know Peter?"

"No, but my very good friend is his very good friend, and he told her to tell me to tell you."

Give me a break. I'm under a lot of stress here, and a neurotically frightened patient has got to do what he's got to do to win friends and influence doctors.

"I think this will help." I hand Dr. Berman the fatal correspondence.

He studies the communiqués. I feel my stomach knotting up, then churning into freefall. If he knows Dr. Upper East Side, he's not saying. He finally finishes reading the letters and places the correspondence in my file. I'm thinking of bad-mouthing Dr. Upper East Side's communication skills (or lack of), but then I think better of it. I don't want my new friend to think I'm a complainer or to violate the relationship doctors have with each other. He turns and approaches.

Where the fuck is Marlowe?

In a careful and deliberate manner, Dr. Berman takes my blood pressure, listens to my heart, and manually examines my abdomen. He wants to know if I have any difficulties urinating: burning, blood, extremely weak streams—the usual suspects.

"No, no, and no."

I confess I'm not coming clean about the loss of the jet stream, a condition I attribute to age, rather than disease. Then it's time for me to turn to my left. I'm so nervous I momentarily lose all sense of direction, something that seems commonplace during these exams. I must remember to bring a GPS with me.

I finally get it right and do as he says. I close my eyes, grab the side of the table with my right hand, and even though Dr. Berman says, "Relax," I tighten up. Grabbing the table isn't the smartest thing, but it's a natural reflex when I think I'm about to be impaled.

The whole thing is over before my knuckles have a chance to turn white. This is unbelievable. I'm in shock as I roll onto my back again and take the box of tissues the good doctor offers me. No pain. *Bupkis*, nothing, *nada, rien*.

He's removing his latex gloves and tossing them in a tall metal waste container. SCORE!

I'm cleaning myself off with a clammy-cold and very unsteady hand. I'm shaking with relief. Okay, maybe a teensy-weensy bit of discomfort, but no pain. No PAIN!

"A little tender, but I don't feel anything abnormal."

I know from previous exams that "abnormal" is code for "bulging with tumors," something none of the other doctors found either. Naturally, I'm reassured to hear my walnut hasn't turned into a five-pointed Star of David.

I think I respond, or maybe the voice I hear is only in my head. Dr. Berman sets up the sonogram machine. I lie back and let him wave his magic wand over my abdomen. It's over in a flash. He instructs me to get dressed. I'm still a little unsteady.

"The sonogram confirms no irregularities."

I'm nodding like a bobblehead.

"Wait here, someone will come in to take blood."

"Sure, sure." I stick my hands under my body to warm them, hoping this will also make them stop shaking.

"Have you left a urine sample?"

"No."

"We'll need one. Then when you're finished, come into my office."

"Okay." My voice is unsteady as my limbs, but thank God he's already halfway out the door and can't possibly hear the shake, rattle and roll.

After Dr. Berman leaves I try to pull myself together. Can it be possible the prostate exam is almost painless? Can it be possible Dr. Berman has magic fingers and my prostate biopsy will also be painless? Can it be possible I have been driving myself crazy for nothing? Can it be possible I have cause for celebration? I don't know whether to cheer or have a migraine.

My problem is solved when the door opens, and in walks the lovely angelic blonde in the pale-blue scrubs who welcomed me when I first came into the office.

"Hello," she says.

"Hello."

"I'm going to take some blood. Is that all right?"

"Sure, sure."

I'm nodding like a bobblehead again, and must stop before I shake my brains loose from their fragile moorings. For a second, I lose my mind and follow Lovely Blonde Nightingale's movements as she prepares the syringe, then I come to my senses and look away.

I point to the chair. "Should I stay here on the table or sit over there?"

"No—where you are is fine."

I hold out both arms. "I have rolling veins. They just discovered it back in September" I want her to know I'm man enough for her.

"Your left arm is the good one."

Damn—I should have worked those biceps. I look away, stare at a blank white space, imagine we're about to kiss. The bloodletting is over before I decide to French her, and guess what—no pain. Okay, I'm feeling a little soreness when I press the cotton down and when she covers it with tape.

Out of the corner of my eye I see Lovely Blonde Nightingale doing something with the vials of my blood. *Don't look. You'll only fixate on the color and imagine all sorts of bad things; how you can think blood looks like transmission fluid defies imagination or anything the Tappett Brothers might dream up.*

"You can get dressed," she says sweetly.

I gingerly let myself down from the table. No hop in my hops now, boys and girls.

"Where can I leave a urine sample?"

"Right across the hall."

She's labeling my vials of blood, something I don't want to watch, and I certainly don't want to interrupt and cause a filing error, but I can't help myself.

"Okay, I'll go right now. Oh, by the way, you were great—absolutely painless; never felt the needle going in or coming out."

No—I'm not looking for brownie points, although it's true I do want them to love me and treat me special. But it's more that it's over—not just the bloodletting, but the entire examination—and I have to blabber—my way of releasing the built-up tension—or else I'll never stop shaking.

I'm going to have to say something to Dr. Berman, too. The Dr. Brown reference only goes so far. But I have to be careful I don't lay it on too thick; calling him "Magic Fingers" is over the top, don't you think?

I slowly dress. My hands are still clammy-cold and a bit shaky-Jakey, but I'm starting to breathe better. I get all my clothes on, check inside my cargo bag to make sure I have all my stuff, and then I head to the head.

The bathroom is tiny. Right away I realize I should have left my stuff in the treatment room, or at least my bulky Hugo Boss coat; what kind of a Fraidy-cat paranoid wouldn't do that? I grab a vial from the three-tier stack of empties, unscrew it, unzip, and wait. This is just like leaving a movie theater, the only other time I have a coat on when I pee.

I'm still unsteady on my feet and unable to wiz on command. I stare up at the little mirror; I'm not as pale as I thought. My hair's a little disheveled, but both my hands are occupied, and I'm not crazy enough to think I can free one without causing serious collateral damage.

Thinking about my hair takes the pressure off (or maybe puts it where it's supposed to be), and I take care of business. I force myself to concentrate, make sure I don't overfill the vial. Not a problem now. My stream's so weak I have time to stop at about the three-quarters mark; not surprising—my walnut's been messed with. Right? Right!

As always, I'm put off by how warm the urine is and I can't wait to put the vial down. Even though giving samples is becoming second nature, I still manage to forget to write my name on the label before I fill up the vial. Fear is the mind-killer and the urine-sample fuck-up. I can't allow my mind to wander into fear overload, or else I'm going to burn out all my circuits and come to a paralyzing stop holding a vial of cooling urine, staring into the bathroom mirror at an aging face I don't want to recognize.

I make sure the vial cap is tight, then I grasp it with one hand, and with the other grab a pen and quickly write *Eric* after where it says *name*, and *Robespierre* under it—perhaps not the correct place to do so, but the damn label is tiny (as usual) and even if there is adequate space, my hand is so shaky I couldn't do it properly. I flush, bring the vial out into the hallway, and Lovely Blonde Nightingale motions me to leave it on the shelf directly to my left. I smile. She smiles. She likes me—I know things about women just the way Clint knows things about birds. I like it when US Secret Service agents are in the house.

I walk over to the reception desk.

"I'm looking for Dr. Berman's office."

"Right there," she smiles, points.

Everyone is smiling here. I pop my head in. Ooops—he's with another patient, so I deftly move back out into the hallway and stand idling next to the reception area; the last thing I want to do is seem pushy. There's a bowl full of candy on the counter. I grab a few, putting two in my pocket and one in my mouth.

Behind me is a huge area full of office people on computers. This is a larger operation than I first thought. I wander over to a spot in the waiting area that still affords me a view of Dr. Berman's door. Not quite James Bond or Jason Bourne, but I do feel the Watchers of MI-5 or Treadstone couldn't really do a better job.

The waiting room is nearly empty and seems surprisingly sadder than when filled with patients. Could it be their lingering aura that provokes this feeling, or am I so in the dumpy-dumps everything seems bleaker?

Finally, a man a little younger than myself leaves Dr. Berman's inner sanctum and approaches the receptionist. He wants to make another appointment. I see this as a signal for me to go in. I cautiously approach the doorway and peek in. Dr. Berman is writing; he looks up and, with a slight wave of a hand, motions me to take a seat. I do as he asks, but I'm at the edge of the chair. Don't misunderstand me, the chair is extremely comfortable, with soft-to-the-touch leather upholstery, but I'm too wired to sit back and relax. Dr. Berman continues to write, so it's either stare at the top of his head or glance around the room. On the wall to my left are framed diplomas and *New York* Magazine Best Doctor awards. On the wall to my right, more awards, under which is a bookcase. On top of the bookcase are nicely framed photographs of Dr. Berman and his family. There are photos of just him with his wife, so photogenic you would think them movie stars or at the very least glamorous socialites. Then there are pictures of the kids (equally photogenic) with and without the parents, and finally, photographs of adorable grandchildren—grandchildren? Again, I'm thinking the guy looks so young.

The number of prestigious medical and post-graduate school degrees plus hospital affiliations are numerous and noteworthy, but it's the *New York* Magazine Best Doctor awards that draw my attention; naturally, I'm still James Bond/Jason Bourne clever, never allowing my gaze to linger should Dr. Berman catch me, think me shallow and just a star fucker. There are more photos on his desk, but they're angled so only Dr. Berman can see them.

He looks up. I grip the sides of my chair.

"If today's blood tests confirm the previous results, I will want to do a biopsy."

If my expression reveals abject horror, he chooses to ignore it. He hands me a sheet that explains the biopsy procedure and how I should prepare for it. The key points: for one week prior to the procedure I am not allowed aspirin or any other medicines that will thin my blood, and the night before, I will need to take an enema. He also writes me out a prescription for an antibiotic I need to take the evening before and for two days following the procedure.

"When should I call you for the results?" I should have cleared my throat. The frogs are croaking!

"The middle of next week," he says, without missing a beat. Obviously toad-talk doesn't throw him off his game.

That's it, then. I extend my hand. "Thank you. I really appreciate your seeing me."

He shakes my hand. "I'll talk to you next week. In the meantime, go out with friends, have a good meal, see a movie."

I clear my throat, nod my head slowly and stand, hoping I have enough balance to get out without swaying. I'm at the door when I remember. I turn.

"By the way, you guys are great here—no pain, nothing." I pat my *tush*.

He nods.

I'm in the hall, in front of the reception desk. The receptionist is smiling at me.

"Do I owe you anything?"

"No, you're all set."

"All right then. Thank you."

I look for Lovely Blonde Nightingale, but I don't see her. I go into the empty waiting room, close up my coat, check to make sure I have everything: glasses, cell phone, keys, wallet. I'm cool.

That's it, then.

I'm out into the street. It's cold and dark.

ROUND 10

FROM the moment my PSA numbers indicate I might have bad walnuts I'm fixating on one thing—THE BIG HURT. Fingers, probes, and most of all—the dreaded biopsy needle. Images of instruments going where none have gone before fill my brain. Then there's the tune that plays over the visuals: Irene Cara is in the house and I can't get her out. Of course, I change the lyrics.

"Pain

I'm gonna have it forever

I'm gonna learn how to cry

I feel it coming together

People will see me and cry

Pain

I'm gonna make it to heaven

Light up the sky like a flame

Pain

I'm gonna have it forever

Baby remember my pain

Remember

Remember

Remember

Remember

Remember

Remember

Remember."

I'm so consumed by my world of hurt there is hardly any time for the real frightener to have an opportunity to spoil my day. Perhaps this is how my brain protects itself? The old neuronal slight of hand: show'em the pain, hide the bad walnuts. What a tricky little devil you are.

I make the necessary phone calls to my kids, making sure I sound upbeat. This is simply a good-sense precaution. A medical double-check, so to speak. *Medical double-check*—I think this is a made-up word, but it flies off my tongue and sounds good, so I use it with both kids. My daughter starts to sob the minute I tell her, and I have to work hard to calm her down. Nick doesn't cry, but I hear his voice catch; *got the Freaky Froggy down there, do you?* They each have tons of questions, and I try to answer them as succinctly as I can while still remaining positive, but with every new question my resolve weakens and I'm having a really difficult time of it. I'm really touched by their sensitivity, and I have to throttle back my own tears, or risk a total breakdown.

I remember dealing with my dad's cancer, and I'm wondering how I can protect my children from experiencing the same sickening dread that numbs the brain, chills the spine, churns the stomach, and ices the limbs. I promise myself I will do everything I can to quell their anxieties by providing up-to-date information, and if the biopsy results are positive for bad walnuts, I will be as optimistic as the results allow me to be. Of course, this will require great acting skills, because my first inclination after receiving bad news will be to find the nearest church steps and crawl halfway up, until with my last breath I utter: *"Is this the end of Ricky?"* *Edward G. is in the house.*

I need reassurance myself, so after I speak to the kids, I call Ira. I again get him at the office and quickly bring him up to date. There's a brief pause, then he assures me there isn't anything to worry about.

"It's a piece of cake."

Good old Ira, sticking to the piece-a-cake story. You would think this would calm me down, and it would if I were a normal person, actually seeking reassurance from someone in the know. Unfortunately, Sir Laurence with a dental drill is in the house.

"Did you feel the biopsy needle? How big was it? They deaden the area before they stick the needle in, don't they? How long did it take? Did you pass out? Were you able to walk afterwards? On a scale of one to ten, ten being the worse, how close to ten was it?"

"Is it safe? Is it safe? Is it safe?"

I put the phone down and stare at the cheap plastic we let pass for high-tech, until I realize I haven't blinked in a minute. I blinkety-blink. This causes either electrical overload, or an epiphany. If the biopsy is truly frightening, the horror would leave an indelible impression and some terror, however small, would still leak out into Ira's consciousness and I would hear clues of it in his voice or words. I didn't—so it isn't.

Whoop-dee-do!

• • •

As I enter Dr. Berman's office, I try to hang on to the *whoop-dee*. I'm also repeating the magic-fingers mantra I've been intoning since I received Dr. Berman's call. It comes just three days after my visit, and I'm caught off-guard. When I see the caller ID, my heart beats so loudly, I'm afraid the neighbors will retaliate by banging on the walls. I don't remember much about the call, certainly not his exact words. I'm surprised he calls me directly and I don't have to wait until a receptionist connects me. Then I remember Dr. Lombardo also made the call himself. Are they just all-around good guys, or is this how they deliver bad news? I do remember his tone is professional, and there's not much I can do but listen, then wait until he puts me through with his receptionist so I can make the appointment. I figure Friday is good, so I will have the weekend to recover. After I make that choice, I become nervous and second-guess myself. Suppose there are complications? It's the weekend, he's away, I'm screwed, but Ira says there won't be any complications. Ira says it's a piece of cake.

I think about taking a bus across 14th to B'way, and then walking down to 9th Street, but that will take thirty minutes, and the less time I have to think about this, the better I'll be, so I take a quick cab over to the office, and here I am.

The waiting room is empty. I take off my coat, hang it up, and bring my cargo bag with me to the reception desk. Lovely Blonde Nightingale comes from the treatment-room area. She's wearing her pale-blue scrubs and looks like she's ready for business.

"Good morning."

"Good morning." She beckons me to follow her. "Do you have anyone to pick you up?"

"Yes, a neighbor." Both my kids want to come, but I know they are working and I don't want to impose. When my neighbor Steve volunteered, I quickly agreed. What a guy.

I enter a treatment room; this one is larger than the last and with more elaborate equipment. She hands me a blue cotton gown.

"Please take everything off except your socks—including your watch and rings. I'll be back in a minute."

I think about saying no.

"Okay."

The room is brightly lit, thanks in part to the sunlight streaming in through the window, and I feel its warming rays as I strip down to my socks. I have trouble figuring out how to put the gown on, until I realize it's just like the one I wear for my colonoscopy; open at the back for quick and easy access. *Whoopee!*

Lovely Blonde Nightingale returns with several release forms for me to sign.

Back out now? Not an option.

"In the last week, have you had any aspirin, drugs, items on the list Dr. Berman gave you that might thin your blood?"

"No."

"Did you take the enema?"

"Yes."

"Did you take the antibiotic this morning?"

"Yes."

"Do you have someone to pick you up?"

Didn't she just ask me that? "Yes."

She checks off my responses. I stare at the forms without reading them, and sign. I'm surprised my hand isn't shaking. This is good. Maybe I can get through this? Lovely Blonde Nightingale puts the forms into my folder, then sets about checking a group of instruments and syringes. I look away.

Dr. Berman enters the room, dressed head to toe in blue scrubs, and I'll be damned if he doesn't look like an alien—not just any ordinary alien, mind you, but a very patrician-like creature. Michael Rennie as Klaatu in *The Day the Earth Stood Still* comes to mind. Come to think of it, even without the scrubs, Dr. Berman does remind me of Michael Rennie. The same chiseled features and tall, lanky frame—why, they could be brothers.

Not so fast, Masked Man! You aren't in movieland anymore, kimosabe. This is real life.

"Good morning, Eric. How are you feeling?"

"Good."

"Did you clean yourself out and take the antibiotic?"

"Yes."

"And, you haven't had any aspirins, blood thinners, any of the products listed on the sheet I gave you?"

"No—I mean, yes, right."

I force a smile. Lovely Blonde Nightingale turns and smiles at me, then returns to her duties.

Dr. Berman explains what's going to happen.

By now you know when I'm in a situation where it's critical for me to pay attention, my DNA reconstitutes itself into that of a highly trained warrior. Skills no normal person possesses kick in. Instructions are three-dimensionally formed, imprinted and remembered pixel by pixel (sort of like what The Terminator could call up in his mind's eye). My brain is so cyborg, years later I will still be able to repeat to the pixel those very same instructions. Right? Right!

"The procedure is going to take about fifteen minutes." He goes on to tell me he will numb the prostate with a topical anesthetic and inject it with Lidocaine. Then he will take core samples from the prostate, which has been divided up into twelve quadrants—one sample from each quadrant, so he doesn't miss anything. "You're just going to feel a little pinch, first from the injection, then from the biopsy needle."

I know from my research that a transrectal ultrasound probe will be used to guide the needle to the correct biopsy location, and that the biopsy is usually done with a spring-loaded needle. (Does this sound like "a little pinch" to you?) The needle quickly enters the prostate gland and removes a tissue sample. (Does this sound like "a little discomfort" to you?) I think they also call this a "punch biopsy." (Since when is a punch a pinch?) Back in the day this was done by hand, now it's all remote control. Well, those magic fingers better know how to operate a joystick, or there'll be no joy in Palookaville today.

To my right I can see the screen of the sonogram machine being maneuvered into position. I don't see the probe or any syringes, but I do see an image on the screen. It's an unshaven, zonked-out Roy Scheider staring red-eyed back at me.

Showtime—and all that jazz . . .

"Before I start, I'm going to give you an antibiotic intravenously."

I nod. This is good. This will prevent infection, a worrisome side effect coming in somewhere between excruciating pain and bleeding to death—entries in a growing list of anything-that-can-go-wrong-*will*-go-wrong that Murphy would be proud of.

As they prepare the intravenous, I'm trying to will myself twenty-four hours into the future, nothing extraordinary as time travel goes. I'm not going very far either, just to my bed at home. I see myself lying there, feeling no unwelcome side effects, perhaps listening to Dinu Lipatti playing a soothing partita for keyboard by Bach, or maybe I'm reading the latest mystery by a favorite author:

Michael Connelly, James Lee Burke, Daniel Silva ... ahh ... *come on, memory, don't fail me now*—John Burdette ... Eliot Pattison—I feel the needle going in, or should I say I imagine the needle going in because I don't feel a thing. I forgot Ian Rankin—how could I have done that?

"Please turn to your left."

Lovely Blonde Nightingale is standing over in that direction and helps me roll over. There is enough play in the IV line so I move over without much trouble.

I'm a little scared, so I try to make a joke.

"I'm a little scared."

So much for me trying to be clever or funny.

"Don't worry, it will be fine," she says, smiling down at me, grinning maybe.

I buy into it. I don't know how my hand gets into hers, but it does, and I'm squeezing as the ultrasound probe is inserted.

"Eric, try to relax."

Okay, maybe you can't call me Sweet Cheeks, but I am trying to muscle down my buttocks; unfortunately, I haven't had any self-control since first grade. You can ask Ms. Caesar—who reigned like Julius, but couldn't rein me—and who made sure I would eventually bend to her demanding desires by following me into the second grade, during which time she became so desperate she sought to break my will by trying to drug me into submission at juice time. (By the way, I always kept one eye open during naptime lest she come by while I was Z-ing and stick a Crayola in my ear.)

Oh, did I tell you, Dr. Berman has this gizmo on his head, some kind of huge magnifying device making him look like a cyclops? Then I'm thinking it comes out of his brain when he's doing surgery, sort of like the creature from *Alien* who likes stomachs as its exit point, but unlike the alien, this gizmo retracts back into Dr. Berman's skull—a third eye so to speak.

Wait, Third Eyes don't have to be sci-fi—they could be Buddhist? Right? Right! I like the idea of something spiritual guiding the ultrasound probe. Maybe that's the source of Dr. Berman's magic fingers ...

"I have to assist Dr. Berman."

Lovely Blonde Nightingale releases my hand. Is this the end of Eric?. ... A healthy body, a healthy body—my kingdom for a healthy body ... Where are those college kids when you need'em? ... And where the fuck is Marlowe? ...

He was in the damn cab, now I can't find him anywhere.

"It'll be fine. You'll feel a little pinch."

This is a signal for my butt cheeks to tighten up. I hope I don't crush the probe. It sounds like a punch, but feels like a pinch. What is this, a question on Jeopardy? Bottom line: bottom is up—and it ain't so bad.

Okey dokey, one down, eleven more to go. I relax.

I hear Dr. Berman give instructions to Lovely Blonde Nightingale. I'm figuring each punch/pinch is followed by the withdrawal of tissue, which then has to be placed in its own individual vial for future lab analysis. This is a proud moment for me—putting this altogether—and a glowing testimonial to the fact my brains aren't up my ass—or if they are, I guess we'll find out soon.

Counting the number of pinches/punches takes all my concentration,, and so I lose count when my mind wanders into Future Toilet Bowl Land, where peeing is painful and bloody.

Pinch—punch—deposit! Pinch—punch—deposit! One—two—cha— cha—cha! I'm getting the hang of it—maybe it isn't so bad—maybe they put something else into the IV besides the antibiotic: a painkiller, muscle relaxers, sedatives? That would account for it. Right? Right!

This is a good thought, and gets me through another series of pinches, punches, and deposits. I'm trying to keep count. Four or five—a quarter of the way through? My math skills are still intact. Maybe I should try doing some square roots? *That's pushing it, Masked Man.*

Two more series of pinches, punches, and deposits, and I'm ready to call it a day. I've reached my level of tolerance. Should I tell Dr. Berman? Perhaps he'd hurry up a bit? Stupid idea. He'll only make a mistake, and then he'd probably have to do the whole freakin' job over again.

"Almost half over, Eric."

Is he reading my mind? What a question, when he's looking up my ass. I let out a sigh. "You're doing a great job."

I think I hear a click. He's making a deposit.

"I'm trying, Dr. Berman, I'm trying."

The trick is to distract yourself, and I'm trying all sorts of things. I'm counting, losing count, trying to remember the count, but my inability to keep things straight just produces frustration. I'm thinking of Lovely Blonde Nightingale and what it would be like to see her lying next to me in bed, naked except for a piece of turquoise jewelry around her neck, smiling, reaching out for my hand and holding it like she did moments ago.

This little mind game gets me through one pinch, punch, and deposit before I do the math and figure I'm old enough to be her grandfather, a sickening thought that jolts me out of this fantasy and forces me to search for something to get me through the next five minutes. Don't ask me where I get the turquoise necklace, that image just pops into my head—and don't get the idea I use jewelry to get women into bed either, because I don't—although I confess, I occasionally play with the notion that if I ever win the lottery, I just might try it on the next Wilhelmina model I meet.

"We're almost finished, Eric."

"Good." What else am I going to say, *Take that pole outta my ass now or I'll beat you over the head with it?* I don't think so.

"Just relax."

"I'm trying."

I'm Marlowe. He is me—I am him.

I wonder if Steve's outside—what time did I tell him? Damn, I can't remember. I hope my kids aren't mad I didn't ask them—they volunteered—that was really nice. I told them I understood how busy they are—Nick's got a freelance shoot, and Gil's got her full-time job. I wonder if Steve's out there already?

AND THEN IT'S OVER! HALLELUIAH!

Hold on, Masked Man—not over yet—can't go home until you pee-pee.

A tech I don't recognize helps me to my feet while Lovely Blonde Nightingale continues to assist Dr. Berman in labeling the twelve samples. I'm wondering if the tech was is in the room the entire time. I'm a little wobbly, but none the worse for wear. I'm not feeling any pain, not even the slightest discomfort. Will this last, or will I be hurting once the drugs wear off?

"Do you want me to urinate now or after I get dress?" I ask Dr. Berman.

"Now."

I knew that would be his answer. Saves me getting undressed again when he puts in the catheter.

"After you're finished, I'd like you to come into my office."

That's a good sign. He must think I'm going to be able to pee.

"Sure—okay, Dr. Berman."

Try to pee when you're afraid you're going to piss out all the blood in your body—it's hell. You've got muscles working against muscles in a tug of war, and only a great force of will decides the outcome.

"Pee, you sonofabitch . . . PEE!"

Here it comes! Thank God no blood, not even a little pink, and no tightness—all right, maybe just a little resistance, but what do you expect after you've had your walnut turned into Swiss cheese? I zip up. I'm relieved beyond measure (no pun intended). The last thing I want is a catheter shoved up my penis; the very thought turns me into a block of ice, and the images of going home with one are just as chilling.

Stop it. It ain't happening, bro, so just wash your hands, and go see Dr. Berman.

On the way to Dr. Berman's office I see Steve. He's reading a magazine and looks up when I appear. I wave.

"I just have to see Dr. Berman. I should be out in little while."

"You okay?"

"Yeah. It wasn't bad at all."

He gives me a thumbs up. My eye goes to a wave of the hand. The guy's got his hat pulled down, but I see it's Marlowe, sitting with his shoulder leaning against the wall, two rows behind Steve. Has he been here the entire time? I knew he was in the cab with me this morning, but when I got out I was totally distracted because I couldn't find the two tens I'm sure I stuck in my coat pocket when I left the house, only to finally find them crumbled up in my jeans after a brief, but frantic search that seemed destined to end in disaster.

Marlowe's nodding. He must be reading my mind. I think I see a smile, but I'm not sure the drugs aren't playing tricks with my eyes.

"I knew you could do it, pally," I swear I hear him say.

I enter Dr. Berman's office. He's changed out of the blue scrubs and into his customary white coat, and no longer looks like a cyclops—but maybe it's the drugs, but damn if he still reminds me of Michael Rennie.

"How do you feel?"

"Fine. I went to the bathroom. No blood, just a tiny bit of tightness."

"Good. You have someone taking you home?"

"Yep."

"I'd like you to stay close to home, relax, order in."

"How long?"

"See how you feel. Monday, if you're up to it, but don't overdo it."

"There's a restaurant at the end of the block."

"That'll be good."

"Any food restrictions?"

"No."

"How about alcohol?"

"Give it a few days. If you have any discomfort, take a nice, warm tub bath. You should also expect some blood and discomfort when you urinate. If you experience more than a little blood, if you have fever or persisting pain, I want you to call me."

"You're around this weekend?"

"Yes. Just call my service."

I stand. I'm sure there are questions I'll regret not asking after I've left, but right now I can't think of anything else. Wait—yes, there is: "How about aspirins? Advil or Aleve?"

"They're fine to take."

I'm out in the hallway. There's an electrifying buzz in the air; the office is filling up. I'm a little wobbly when I go up to the desk and grab a handful of candies.

"They're good, aren't they, pally?"

"Yes, they are."

His eyes are fluttering under the fedora, as soundless as the oscillation of butterfly wings to a deaf man. I can't believe no one asks him to take the sinister-looking thing off. He puts a callused hand on my shoulder. It feels good to be alive.

ROUND 11

IT'S impossible to know how you're going to cope with the waiting, but one thing is certain, when pain (as in, the fear of) is a magnificent obsession, waiting is a bitch. I take it back, I don't want to use the word *obsessed*—rather, I would like to think of myself as *concerned*, which speaks to a healthier state of mind. Obviously, I'm most fixated during the first hours after the punch-out, and I pay strict attention to any slight deviation in my health. I'm tired, but I'm sure most of my fatigue is due to stress, which is only natural. I'm avoiding anything strenuous, but I have to get in and out of the cab, go up to my apartment, change into sweatpants, all of which I accomplish at a snail's pace; the good news is there is no pain and just the tiniest of soreness when I sit in the wrong position, which I discover is any position that puts too much pressure on my *tush*. Dr. Berman warns me this may be a side effect and suggests warm baths, perhaps two or three a day to relieve the soreness.

So—what's the big problemo? Peeing, or more to the point, peeing blood until I faint dead away. I know there's no way I can bleed to death, but clearly logic plays a secondary role to my neurosis. In Dr. Berman's office my urine is clear, the first time at home it's reddish/pinkish. From then on it's an off-again, on-again occurrence, and each visit to the bathroom devilishly plays with my head. Clear, and I'm singing "Sweet Sue." Anything less, and I'm singing the blues.

During the first day, I'm either lying on the couch watching TV, or on my bed, dozing. I'm by myself most of Friday, except for when Steve comes down. He's on his way out and wants to know if I need anything. On Saturday, Gillian comes over, and on Sunday Nick and his wife, Jen, visit. The scenarios are the same. They come for lunch (we order in), and shortly afterwards they leave. This is perfect, because I'm really tired, though it's more mental fatigue than physical wear and tear. Sure, my body is recovering from the pinching and punching, but it's the stress from trying to stay positive that's really the killer.

Family visits are good, because they remind me of how strong my father was during his battle with cancer, and I vow to be just as resolute. It was only at the very end that my father wavered, and then it was only to wonder why, when things were going so well for him, he had to get sick. This was one of the worst moments for me, and I almost lost it, but somehow I remember I forced the tears back until I left the living room where we had put the hospital bed and went into the bathroom so a flushing toilet covered up the avalanche of sobs.

Unfortunately, being with the kids also forces me to see the fear that flickers in their eyes when I catch their sideway glances. I try not to lock eyes, usually breaking the gaze with a smile and a joke. I want to get up and hug them, tell them everything is going to be all right, but I would be turning into a jumping jack, and that kind of impulsive behavior would only make everyone more anxious.

My daughter-in-law is a human reality check, because she asks the medical questions the kids dare not to. Jen was the same when she and the kids visited my dad when he was in the hospital in Atlantic City. The first thing she did was to go to the medical chart that hung at the foot of his bed and began to read it. The kids were crouched around the bed; Gillian may even have been sitting on it, so my dad couldn't see Jen, but I could, and I motioned for her to put the chart back before my father could ask her what it said. I was being overly protective, because my father left all the questions up to me, and it was only when we were alone that I could bring him up-to-date, usually relaying such innocuous details as his temperature or fluid intake—not only for the reasons that I didn't want to frighten him, but because the doctors' stories were muddled and I hadn't the foggiest idea what was draining the life out of him. That visit would be the second-to-last time they saw him alive.

Today, I welcome Jen's questions, because it affords me the opportunity to give a blow-by-blow account of the biopsy (excepting my Lovely Blonde Nightingale fantasy and the bathroom peeing scene). This is not new. I enjoy providing detailed narratives, sometimes so descriptive my information can border on the boring, but I keep a watchful eye on my audience, and if attention strays and they become fidgety, I skip the small stuff, stick to the essentials, and with dramatic flare speed up the story. This usually does the trick, and gives another meaning to the popular saying, *The devils in the details.*

I'm having no such problem today. The story of my biopsy holds everyone's attention, and the fact it went so painlessly and without any major side effects (knock on wood, let's keep it that way) fills everyone in the room with a great sense of relief and perhaps a sense of hope that my biopsy will show no evidence of cancer. I give Jen an extra-tight hug. If she hadn't asked the questions my children were afraid to ask, I'm not sure I would have had the courage to tell my story. Everyone is all laughter and smiles when they leave, and I think if my enthusiastic chronicle can give voice to this optimism, perhaps it will also become a self-fulfilling prophecy—and if that's the case, I can't wait to tell all my friends the story.

I decide to watch the entire *Brideshead Revisited* epic. It's an eleven-episode series, a 660-minute presentation—or so it says on the back of the digitally remastered collector's edition DVD box. It's not entirely for my benefit, but also for my lovely guest. I get the idea to watch the show while I'm dozing and Jeremy Irons, Anthony Andrews, and Diana Quick appear to me in a dream. Lovely Blonde Nightingale is with them, dressed as they are in the elegant, but casual attire of their class and time, and looking not the least bit out of place. I suspect Lovely Blonde Nightingale has more than a bit of English in her, and I must remember to ask her the next time I see Dr. Berman.

When I wake I'm also hungry, and find a roast turkey sandwich with lettuce, tomato, and mustard on a semolina hard roll. Lovely Blonde Nightingale clinically examines all the local markets for fresh turkey, finding many pretenders until hitting upon the real thing at Bruno the Ravioli King. After all, she is a nurse, and wants to make sure I'm eating healthily, and not adding unnecessary calories to an already slightly overweight body. I'm happy a woman is here to look after me, even if she's still in her pale blues.

Normally, I'm ashamed of my digs, a place still furnished with my father's 50s furniture and faux-antique carpet remnants, cram-jam with my books, VCR tapes and *New Yorker* Magazines on bookshelves, table tops, and stacked under all available cabinets. Everywhere you look there is no escaping these dust collectors—not quite a Collyer Brothers mansion, but still an eyesore, and certainly no stately pleasure-dome decree. *To this you invite a woman of exquisite earthly beauty and divine grace, who most certainly has royal blood racing through her Rule-Britannia body? I don't think so.* The sandwich is really dry and could use mayo.

I usually have a two-pound bag of Epsom salts sitting next to the tub, and liberally pour the stuff in when I'm soaking my aching body—not that it's medically proven to work, but like the best talking-myself-into-it-placebo, I always find instant magic-potion gratification, only today I don't dare use it, thinking the stuff will cause bodily harm. I'm totally ignorant of the laws of canonical quantum gravity and human physiology, or else I would know there is no way the stuff can get sucked up Mr. Floppy and into my walnut—nevertheless, when in fear, let your neurosis rule. (One bodily function I understand.) I could ask Lovely Blonde Nightingale, but why draw attention to my ignorance instead of allowing it to tantalizingly show itself during the normal course of the relationship, like a stripper slowly removing her clothes instead of shedding them in one rip of a breakaway costume.

Just as Dr. Berman predicts, the soaking relieves the soreness, but now I'm obsessing over whether or not the heat will cause me to bleed more. Hold on, I'm not bleeding in the first place—and in the second place, if a hot soak can make the walnut bleed, why would Dr. Berman prescribe it in the first place? *Ahh-ha, Masked Man!* The light bulb flickers in the dimness of my brain!

Lovely Blonde Nightingale's appreciation for architecture, interior design, fashion, and cinematography is surprisingly in sync with mine, and we find ourselves gushing and gawking at the same scenes as they flash upon the screen. She also loves the unforgettable theme music, and when I point out the magnificent prose, she will then ask me to pause the recording and go back so we can hear the narration a second time, something I do frequently when I'm watching shows like *Brideshead Revisited.* I keep thinking I'm going to purchase the book so I can follow the film, like one does with an opera libretto. One day I will try it, although I'm sure Waugh's book is nothing like the teleplay, and probably makes the libretto idea unworkable.

There is no question that having a loved one around during a health crisis—any crisis, for that matter—is a gift, and should be cherished; the sustenance provided is life-giving, life-affirming, and the best medicine I could get at this time. Having someone in the house is new to me, and I must admit, I can get a little cranky when my routine is interrupted by another's needs, or when certain rules applying to good apartment living are broken, no matter how ethereal the visitation. I'm speaking now of Lovely Blonde Nightingale's white clogs, which make such a clatter on the bare wooden floors that I'm afraid they disturb my downstairs neighbor. I solve the problem for myself by walking around in socks or bare feet. I hear that's good for the body; however, I really do it because I'm too cheap to purchase carpeting, although I still have my father's small area rugs, one of which is strategically positioned in the bedroom where noise is most offensive.

I mention the clogs to Lovely Blonde Nightingale, who assures me she's light-footed and her footsteps couldn't possibly be heard below; unfortunately, she has terrible arches, and needs to wear these clogs, or else she'll have severe shooting pains, a condition she developed during nursing school and one that has just gotten worse over the years. I have yet to inquire why she's still in her scrubs, and I'm not sure I will, because I can clearly see questioning her footwear was totally uncalled for. All that matters is she's here, sitting beside me on the couch watching Jeremy Irons confronting his aloof father, played by Sir John Gielgud, during one of their dinning scenes, a moment made so tense by the father's cold and remote personality that I squirm, I fidget in sympathy for the unfortunate son, and for one exquisite moment I completely forget my pierced walnut or that I may have cancer. (There, I said it!)

As we continue our *Brideshead*-marathon weekend, scene stealer Nickolas Grace doing his outrageous portrayal of the flamboyant sybaritic flamer Anthony Blanche, complete with the most memorable and clearly enunciated stutter, sends us both into hysterics. And when he orders and drinks those two White Russians, our mouths water, but finally, after some soul searching, we come to the conclusion that going out to a bar and getting soused on these chocolate delights wouldn't be best for my recently abused gland or her unblemished nursing reputation.

On Monday, I'm totally alone, but I decide taking the elevator down to the main floor to get my mail is absolutely doable. I'm walking crab-like, as if normal motoring will rip those twelve neatly placed punch holes. I imagine a punctured water hose spraying a dozen thin streams of blood into the air, drenching the green lawn and turning it into a mud-soaked field of red. These images change as I approach my elevator, replaced by the blood pouring out of the elevator scene in The *Shining*. "*Redrum, redrum, redrum . . .* "

The door opens and Erica, my upstairs neighbor, stands right there in front of me. Her proximity to the door momentarily catches me off guard, but her great big smile and hello immediately puts me back on my game. I hope she hasn't heard my mumblings.

"Hi, how are you?" I ask.

"Pretty good. And you?"

"I'm good."

"Good."

"Oh, you didn't hear anything last night, did you? I mean, I have my father sleeping over and we were walking around late last night."

"No, I didn't hear a thing. I never hear anything—you're really a considerate neighbor."

"Thanks. You are, too."

"Thanks."

She's looking at me, smiling, and suddenly, I'm thinking this crazy stuff: *Do I look different? Do I look like I just had twelve pieces of tissue punched out of my walnut? Do I look pale from leaking blood every time I pee?*

I'm only wearing a fleece pullover, so when I open the outer door, a blast of cold air hits me square in the chest and I quickly get myself back into the lobby. The mailbox is empty, and I think I should stop being so damn cheap, and get myself a subscription to Netflix. Why an empty mailbox should trigger images of that little red envelope is beyond me, unless flying under the radar in my unconscious air space, *redrum*s are still snapping away at my synapses.

I ride an empty elevator back to my floor, and when my eye wanders up to the security camera I want to announce to those watching: *Hey, what are you staring at? I'm not sick. You don't have to pity the old guy with bad walnuts.*

I'm thinking back to last night and my conversation with Ira. His call came after those from Ellyn and Helen. I'm thankful I've got friends who care about me. I'm also sure their messages of hope contribute to my feelings of well-being (they call every day), although my first reaction to their good cheer is to turn my eyes toward the dark side.

What the hell is wrong with me?

Ira's message is hard to contradict, so I don't: He has been through it. It worked for him and so far, as he predicted, it's working for me. I give him the report and we compare experiences. He doesn't remember Lovely Blonde Nightingale, and he certainly doesn't mention taking her home with him to watch *Brideshead* (Sharon would kill him), so I leave that part out. I want to know how he dealt with the waiting.

"I was working. I didn't have time to think about anything else but my business."

I'm working, too. I'm playing around with two ideas for novels: one about a three-hundred-pound woman in her forties from a whacky and highly dysfunctional, morbidly obese Italian family, whose life changes dramatically after gastric bypass surgery; the other the reincarnation of the famed Queen of the Nile, who enlists the help of an Internet-dating guru to locate her long-lost Anthony, whose aura she has detected on the Van Wyck Expressway while traveling into the Big Apple from Kennedy on her yearly visit to the Temple of Dendur at the Met. I re-read both, and while I'm happy with the writing (and the distraction it causes), I no longer have passion for either one, and decide to temporarily put them aside and, instead, decide to write about my prostate. But I don't have much enthusiasm for this subject, either, so what's the deal here? Any extraordinary experiences that make my story unique? No. Brilliant medical or psychological insights? Double no. Unique battleground (outer space, vampire crypt)? I only wish. A huge fan base hanging onto my every move? Wouldn't that be nice? No—I'm doing this because during my dream weekend, a little voice crept into my brain chatter and told me: *Eric, put your troubles in your old kit bag and write, write, write.*

Ironic—escaping your worries by writing about them. Then I'm thinking of *Crime and Punishment* and *The Brothers Karamazov*, two of the best psychological thrillers of all time and, like all of Dostoevsky's writings, examples of how the author is struggling with his own loss of faith and using this medium to work it all out. I'm no Melville expert, so I can't talk about *Moby Dick*, but certainly Kafka, Camus, and Sartre also make my point. I'm just hoping I come to a better end than Camus who, upon reflection, unconsciously influences my opening paragraph, which comes easily (*quelle surprise*)—and before I know it, I'm twenty pages in by the time my Friday appointment with Berman rolls around (more surprising), and I'm wondering where the hell this writing voice comes from.

Writing about my present-day woes strikes me as embarrassingly egotistical, and on top of that boring, so my first inclination is to ignore an autobiography, but this style eventually wins out. I suspect this enthusiasm may be misplaced rebellion, but nevertheless I quickly become absorbed in my work to the point that I'm only fixating on my troubles a third of my waking moments, and best of all, I discover I've got lots to say and am liking how I'm saying it.

"Mr. Robespierre, Dr. Berman will see you now."

I look up. Lovely Blonde Nightingale is nowhere to be seen. I suspect she's in with a patient, although I haven't spotted her since I arrived. Maybe it's her day off? It's another tech who calls my name, pronouncing it perfectly and with just a hint of a Spanish accent.

I'm back in the biopsy room and I get a rush. *I'm done with that sucker, my man.* I realize this new tech is a young Hispanic, no more than twenty-five. She wants to take my blood pressure. She smells deliciously of roses and I'm more than happy to let her do anything as long as she stays close.

"It's one-thirty-four over eighty-seven," she tells me.

"I'm usually one-twenty over eighty."

"Did you just get here?"

"Yep."

"You're probably still out of breath."

My lying lips say, "Sure, that's it," but my paranoia says *high blood pressure.*

"Dr. Berman will be in shortly."

"Okay."

When Dr. Berman enters, I'm up on the table still sniffing, lost in romantic visions of Nurse of Aromatic Delight running naked through an overgrown rose garden. I'm also dangling my feet, which are swinging freely to a beat only my subconscious can hear. I stop, embarrassed. I hope he doesn't think I have Saint Vitus Dance. He goes right to my chart.

"How are you feeling?"

"Fine. For the first few days I had a little blood in the urine, not all the time, but now it's totally clear; a little soreness every so often, but that usually goes away after a long soak—other than that I'm okay."

I don't think I should tell him about the blood in the semen, how painful my ejaculations are, or how afraid I am to try it again; confessing this might lead to blabbing about Lovely Blonde Nightingale.

"Lie on your back and undo your pants."

"Okay."

I unzip and lie back. Quickly, and as efficiently as always, Dr. Berman manually examines my abdomen and then runs the sonogram wand over it. If I have bad walnuts, I can't tell it from his demeanor, so either I'm going to have to ask, or wait until he decides it's time to give me the test results.

He's saying something about this examination. "Everything seems to be fine."

He wants me to get dressed and come into his office. That's it, then. It's decided. I'll wait until he tells me. There is never a choice. I simply don't have the *cojones* to ask. Dr. Berman pats me on the shoulder and leaves me with a smile. I'm fucked! Why else would he show that much personal kindness—because he's feeling sorry for me, that's why, boys and girls. Next thing he'll be asking me to pay in advance.

I think about never leaving this room. I think about just putting on my clothes and walking out the front door. But I decide to grow an extra set and head toward his office.

Dr. Berman turns a sheet of paper around so I can see it. It's a picture of my walnut, divided up into quadrants, twelve of them—pinched and punched within some of those quadrants tiny circles—some empty, some filled and looking like phases of the moon—and that's when I know—or it may be because Dr. Berman tells me—CANCER . . .

The moon-like circles pull me in. Suddenly, I'm drawing an imaginary line from one to another, creating a constellation—an astrological sign—the unmistakable outline of a skeleton lowered into the ground. I'm not shaking, I'm not soiling my pants, I'm calmly listening to Dr. Berman explain what he found, what it means, and what options are open to me. I'm glad Nick and Gil aren't here. I'm not sure I could handle their emotional response, although I *could* use a hand to hold. When I finally look up at Dr. Berman, the familiar Marlowe profile and sudden flicker of eye movement under the grey fedora appears in the window, the solitary figure momentarily stooping as if bending to tie an open shoelace.

"Don't worry, pally—I got more holes in me than that, and I'm still standing."

Then the shamus is gone, and I'm listening to Dr. B.

Dr. Berman covers the first sheet with a blank one. He angles the paper so I can see it.

GRADE 1–5
3
score 3 + 4 = 7
4 (in a circle)
2–10 (range)

"This is the Gleason scale, and you have a moderate grade in the early stages."

Moderate—that's a good word—good enough to reduce my heartbeat by a few hundred miles per hour.

STAGING
PSA = 4.1
(arrow down)
10;
DRE = NL;
0/0 + (circled)
BX = LOW/VOL (in a box)
BONE SCAN (bone circled)
CT (circled)
TREATMENT
WATCHFUL WAITING
LOWFAT DIET (crossed out)
CRYOSURGERY – LACK OF DATA (underlined)
SURGERY (two lines leading to:)
INCONTINENCY 5% (circled)
BLEEDING – TRANSFUSION RECUPERATION.
I'm shaking my head.
RT (lines leading to:)
EXT and SEEDS (lines leading to:)
8 1/2 weeks
(circle with little squibs in them indicating the seeds that will be implanted)
(lines leading to:)
IRRITATIVE, MEDICATION, ERRECTILE DYS (underlined)
I'm nodding. "That's what I want."
CHEMO – PALLIATIVE/EXP
HORMONAL (lines leading to:)
ADJUCTIVE (circled) and PALLATIVE

I'm out on the street. So this is what it's like to have cancer?

And what feeling is that, Mr. Robespierre? Do you actually feel any different?

It's a real winter evening in the big city, the temperature around thirty-two degrees, with a wind gusting to close to fifty miles an hour, making it bone chilling when the wind smacks you—and that happens when I hit Broadway.

Would you feel any different if you didn't have cancer?

Fuck, yes! It would be Aruba Time, baby!

Actually, it's almost a relief in a strange way, because when the last element of doubt is removed, so is all the stress it took to hold onto that positive attitude. In a way, hedging my bet and thinking the worse paid off—because when my most terrible fears become a reality, it's no surprise to my ass, and I don't want to jump in front of a subway train.

I want a glass of red wine, but I hate drinking without eating and I hate eating alone. It's too late to call Steve and I'm not sure I want to sit down with my kids while I do scenes from *The Lost Weekend* or *The Days of Wine and Roses*.

I'll call the kids, but not while I'm walking, although I do always see those die-hard Chatty Cathys freezing their hands and faces off as they scream into their cell phones and into the howling wind, their collective voices caught up in the swirling vortex hurling through the canyons of lower Manhattan.

I'm over to Fourth Avenue, and as I walk one block north, I keep coming back to my surprising state of mind. I see a pattern emerging: periods of anxious speculation feeding upon itself, threatening to eat me up alive, followed by The Knowing that now translates to bad walnuts—prostate cancer, early stages, moderate grade—a prognosis imprinting itself like a potent tranquilizer, settling my brain chemicals, turning down the levels of ferocity from Hulk Hogan to Cool Hand Luke.

I decide to stop at Bruno's the Ravioli King for two slices and a bowl of *pasta e fagioli*, which I will buy right after purchasing a bottle of Jacob's Creek Cabernet from the liquor store across the street—*not* the other way round, something I have mistakenly done; that ends up making the take-out even colder. Sure, I could heat it up in the micro, but pizza is never the same when you do that, and it robs the flavor from the soup, too.

Everybody else apparently also has pizza on the brain, so I have to wait on a long, noisy line, but I'm in better shape than the frozen souls who are shivering uncontrollably, mostly doctors, nurses, and techs from Beth Israel, who come across First Avenue in only their flimsy blue and green scrubs. I search their young faces, looking for those who stare back at me, the mark of those who can pick a cancer victim out of any line-up, anytime, anywhere, even when freezing and overwhelmed by the powerful tomato-ey aroma of pizza and *pasta e fagioli*. But they're busy chatting:

"I'm seeing Jimmy, but his hours are worse than mine."

"What do you think about Jamaica? You know, the same place Kara went."

"Oh, I saw her pictures."

"I had to access the shunt insertion site, but there wasn't any infection."

"Whatever happens, I'm not going back to Boston."

I escape without anyone giving me so much as a nod, and make it home before I smother myself with the scarf I've tied tightly over my nose and mouth. A trio of college kids exits my building as I come in, so busy lighting up or turning on cell phones that they fail to hold open either door. The outer door isn't a problem, but the inner one requires a key, so I have to put the food and wine packages down, or else risk turning the pizza over, or opening up the soup container and losing half its contents, something that's ninety-percent guaranteed based on previous bouts of laziness that overwhelmed my better angels—simple everyday inconveniences, the minutiae of living that I realize I stand to miss if the cancer gets me.

Soon I'm sitting in front of the TV, watching an old "CSI" on Spike, when this maudlin piece of insight lights up my left hemisphere like a flash grenade. (Coincidence? I think not!) William Petersen, the star of the show—who I've liked ever since *Manhunter* and the even better *To Live and Die In L.A.,* the Friedkin masterpiece that features a car chase going against traffic (a first, and one copied many times, even by Friedkin himself in the equally masterful *Ronin*)—is giving testimony in court during a time of intermittent deafness, the exposure of which would send his character, Gil Grissom, into early retirement. Naturally he wins the day, and at the end of the scene signs to his nemesis who had hopes of ruining Peterson. This is a great gotcha moment, as well as a dramatic device to make certain even the dumbest of viewers get the fact that he's lip read his way out of a jam.

Well, it's the lip reading that sets off the flash grenade, bringing back the moment in time just after Dr. Berman tells me I have an 85% chance of full recovery—he casually, but matter-of-factly informs me I will need to have a CT and full bone scan to make sure the cancer is contained (he's confident it is). This is when I go deaf *à la* Petersen, and find myself lip reading, "CT and full bone scan." Ordinarily, total loss of hearing would send me up the wall, but I'm preoccupied with images of tiny cancer cells hiding in my organs, round little fuckers with smiley faces, looking up at me like I see Grissom look at his nemesis: *GOTCHA!*

Done in by the day's events and the two glasses of red, I fall asleep on the couch and wake to another episode. I'm watching a tape marked *"CSI" Marathon II,* so I can't tell from looking at the screen how many episodes I've missed, but the clock on the cable box reads 9:30 p.m., so I'm thinking an hour and a half's worth, maybe. I'm so headachey, I'm not sure of anything except that Lovely Blonde Nightingale is next to me, sleeping, her head comfortably resting on two pillows she got from the bedroom and stacked on top of the sofa, something I first saw her do during our *Brideshead* fest, and an idea that never came into my head in all the years of falling asleep in front of the TV. I detect the slightest snore, more like a purr, and I think of my own horrible snoring, which frequently becomes so disturbing it even wakes me. I think of the times my ex-wife/girlfriends jab, poke, shake me awake—certainly a better alternative than smothering me with a pillow, a choice I'm sure crosses their minds (it would mine), a choice a murder jury would be sympathetic to, probably rendering an innocent plea even before lunch is served.

I don't want to wake Lovely Blonde, Nightingale, but it's also against my nature to leave the TV or the lights on, so I turn both off, and fortunately my actions don't disturb my ghostly visitor. I leave the hall light on so she can find her way to the bedroom. I also cover her thin scrubs with a second Afghan— she's already is using the red checked one from the couch, but it doesn't cover her shoulders, and the yellow-and-black wooly I get from the closet is perfect for that.

My head is swimming and I know I need to sleep, but I'm tempted to wake her, tell her what Berman told me, hopefully get her to tell me I have nothing to worry about. But I think better of it. so I wash my face, brush my teeth, take an Aleve, strip down to my shorts and a tee and hit the sack—but just before that I take a fairly long and semi-strong wiz and hope I'll be able to sleep halfway through the night, because the last thing I want to do is wake up every three hours and find that during one of these bathroom visits my worries will prevent me from going back to sleep, forcing me to see those smiley faces and hear "GOTCHA!" over and over until the dawn breaks and I'm totally wiped and fried.

I call Ira the next evening and tell him about my meeting with Dr. Berman. I know he's gotten the radiation and the seeds, but I don't remember him telling me about the hormone shots.

"Yep, I got them."

"I'm supposed to get two: one before the radiation, the second between the radiation and the seed implants."

"I don't remember, but I think I got more than that. I have to ask Sharon."

"Any side effects from the hormones?"

He tells me to buy high heels. I tell him I already got in touch with my feminine side and bought a pair, plus some nice chiffon dresses he can borrow if he's nice to me. I say we should go bra shopping, but I stop myself from mentioning nipple rings. We laugh it up, and for a moment I'm relieved I haven't lost my sense of humor; unfortunately, my mood changes back to *serioso* when I tell him Dr. Berman is sending me for CT and bone scans.

"Dr. Berman sent me, too. It's normal procedure. Don't worry about it."

Ira's confident my cancer has not spread. I'm not so sure, but I don't elaborate or share with him my off-and-on-again back pain, which my MRI says comes from a herniated disk; I've seen *The Shootist*—I remember how the same symptoms put the Duke six feet under.

I bring up the radioactive issue, specifically that Dr. Berman told me I would have to use a condom during sex, and if I'm sleeping with a woman, we need to have a couple of pillows separating us.

"He never told me that."

"Well, he told me. Obviously, he figures me for a wild and crazy stud and you for an old, married geezer."

"Dr. Burson. my oncologist, didn't say anything, either."

"I haven't seen Dr. Burson yet. I think I meet him after my scans. Dr. Berman told me children and pregnant women can't sit on my lap."

"They both told me that, too. What about you and me? Of course, I'd be in my blue chiffon dress."

We laugh. There it is—another feminine (gay) reference, behind which experts say lie a multitude of homophobias. These references remind me of something else—an article describing how too much testosterone causes prostate cancer; does that mean it's either becoming gay or getting cancer? I realize how idiotic and scientifically untrue this is. Not all gay men have low levels of T, and not all straights are brimming full of it, either. Bad walnuts are an equal opportunity fuck-you—that's all there is to it.

Ira has to jump (another meeting outside the office), but first we plan on dinner for sometime next week.

I'm feeling better when I head into the kitchen. Ira's success is a serious confidence booster—could the warm and fuzzies be close behind?

As coincidence would have it (or does he call her?), Ellyn rings me two minutes after I hang up with her brother-in-law. We catch up, and it's clear she agrees with Ira—the prognosis is good and the tests just precautionary.

"I was in your neighborhood last night," Ellyn mentions.

"Where?"

"Butai."

"I know it."

It's the newest of the trendy Flatiron-area restaurants, and just a couple of blocks west of me. In fact, a week or two ago Steve and I saw the place for the very first time.

Every window table is filled with gorgeous women. *Look, they're waiting for us.* Steve is directly dialed into the singles scene, so when he presses his cold nose up against the window (picture a drooling kid peering into FAO Schwarz at Christmas time) and smiles at the blonde in the red dress just inches away, I follow his lead—and suffer real shame when she turns away without as much as giving us a second look, a move that only makes Steve bow with *beau geste* gusto. I can only marvel at his flare, and picture Gary Cooper striking a similar pose. Naturally, I'm not going to relay this story to Ellyn.

"Butai is a 'robata' restaurant."

"Huh?"

"In Japanese, 'robata' means 'by the fireside,' and refers to the centuries-old, country-style cooking of northern Japanese fishermen."

"Thank you, Mamma San Julia Child."

Ellyn's description of the dishes make my mouth water: butter-sautéed potato pancakes; shrimp, lotus root and shiso tempura wrap; main dishes like grilled whole shelled jumbo prawns with sea salt; organic chicken seasoned with sea salt; and sides like sliced pork belly with daikon and ponzue sauce; Japanese yam potato; and pumpkin with sweet yakitori sauce.

As she talks, I rummage around in my refrigerator looking for something Japanese until I settle on the product with the only remotely foreign sounding name in my fridge: a strawberry Activia. I finish up this woeful substitute in two teaspoonfuls, while Ellyn mercifully ends her food review.

We discuss lunch plans. She's up in Greenwich, but she's coming into the city two weeks from today to have dinner with her daughter, so we make a date and agree to go to Butai, her treat.

I imagine the fishermen who originally lived and cooked in what they now refer to as "old world" Japan—strong, healthy men leading strong, healthy lives. I wonder if their very distant progeny, grandsons of grandsons of grandsons, now my age, have dreams of killing their fathers?

Within the next hour, both my kids call. I give them each the good-news version, leaving out the CT and bone scan to spare them—and me—the anxiety. Nick and Gil are relieved, and want to know more about the radiation and seed implantation.

"I'm getting more info next time I meet with the doctor."

They don't press me for the date, and I don't tell them, because I know it won't be happening until the results of the scans are in, and that won't happen until a week from today.

Nick wants to come by for lunch tomorrow. He's got to go into the office in the morning, but then he'll drive by to pick me up. He has a packet of info on prostate cancer his upstate neighbor gave him for me. From what Nick tells me, the guy underwent treatment two years ago and appears to be one-hundred-percent A-okay, and Nick says the same will happen to me.

After I finish with the kids, I'm staring at a rerun of "Law and Order: Criminal Intent," and it dawns on me that there's got to be something special about Fridays, because it seems all my tests and procedures are happening on that particular day of the week. Sam's suddenly in the house, and I'm cookin' with Cooke.

"Another Friday night and I ain't got nobody
I've got some worries 'cause I just seen the doc
Now, how I wish I had someone to talk to
I'm in an awful way
I got the numbers a month ago
I seen a lot of girls since then

If I could meet 'em I could get 'em
But as yet I haven't met 'em
That's how I'm in the state I'm in
Another Friday night and I ain't got nobody
I've got some worries 'cause I just seen the doc
Now, how I wish I had someone to talk to
I'm in an awful way"

I wake up every three hours to pee, and while I used to bitch and moan about this inconvenience, tonight I'm just happy there's no pain, no blood, and I can hear the sweet steady sound of my water hitting the toilet water. This happiness carries me back to my bed on winged feet (the bad poet made me say it), and before I know it, it's 8:30 a.m. and I'm up and fully rested.

Sam's lyrics are still running through my head. I hope he doesn't come down from heaven and smack me because I fooled around with his words.

Nick shows up at 12:30 p.m., and when he sees I'm looking and acting like I'm a hundred percent, he feeds on my optimism and we head downtown to Lucky Strike, two guys rocking and rolling to the bluesy melodies of Mississippi Fred McDowell on the stereo.

"When the train come along, Lord
When the train come along, Lord
Gonna meet her at the station
When the train come along
If you see my mother
And she ask for me, Lord
Gonna meet her at the station
When the train come along
(guitar)
When the train come along, Lord
When the train come along, Lord
Gonna meet her at the station
When the train come along
If you see my father
And he ask for me, Lord
Gonna meet him at the station
When the train come along"

"Nothing like a song about death to perk up your day," I say to him, and then I see his face. "Oh, sorry. I'm just kidding, Nick. Keep it on, it's a great tune."

Many a jest is said in truth, but I keep that to myself and stop with this sorry business. Remember, cancer means never having to say you're sorry. (So, is this any cheesier than the original?). Who the hell takes lyrics to a song seriously? Yeah—right. Strip music lyrics from my brain and I'm left with movie lines and comic routines; that's a third of my intellect gone, not to mention say goodbye to singing in the shower or along with the radio, no more "peaceful, easy feeling" in my life.

Both my kids love music, and naturally they're into their own music, but they still have a deep affection for the tunes I exposed them to during their childhood and remember the songs I played on long car rides up to our house in Connecticut, and still talk about the moments they fell in love with CCR, The Eagles, Bob Seger, and countless other rockers and doo-woppers from the Fifties and Sixties.

It was raining when I got into Nick's Nissan SUV, and the forecast is for more of the same, maybe even some snow. Who cares if it's a cold, dreary day? I love driving around the city on the weekends when you can zip around, if you catch the lights right, go great distances, say from 96th Street to 42nd without seeing one red light. Like back in the day, when there were just a third of the cars and cabs you see today; the only trouble with weekends is the unexpected street closing (thy name is fucking street fairs).

Lucky Strike is down in Soho, on Grand off West Broadway. On the way we drive through the East Village, the Bowery, and then west over to Soho, neighborhoods full of unique and interesting architecture, cityscapes where you can still look up and see the sky. I'm having a great time, and for the moment forget I'm transporting cells that seek to destroy me, cells I gave birth to, but now have turned against the one who continues to give them life—a good life, I might add.

The ungrateful buggers—why I oughta . . .

Hello—Mr. Wallace Beery is in the house, raising a threatening hand to Jean Harlow (*Dinner at Eight,* or was it *China Seas?*)

Just as we come around Grand, we notice the brake lights of a jet-black 911 flick on and hear the turbo rev up. What luck—right across the street from the restaurant. We give him a thank-you wave and he gives us a you're-welcome toot in return. The throaty roar of his super-charged rocket makes my testosterone boil, and I'm thinking, *Will this kill the cancer?* The noise ricochets through the deserted street, reverberates with a vengeance against the tin and brick facades of imposing, block-long, turn-of-the-century structures, many designated landmarks, one more magnificent than the next. I swear I can feel the ground shake under the Nissan's tires. Nick and I look at each other.

"Cool . . . "

"Cool . . . . "

Before we get out, Nick hands me a large manila envelope.

"Here's the stuff Frank Rivera gave me. It's a lot of research, plus stuff his doctors and hospital gave him. If you have any questions, he wants you to call him—the number's on the back of the envelope."

I'm overwhelmed by the gesture. I hug Nick just before we enter the restaurant. I have another reason for wanting to see my son today: I have something important to talk to him about. Nick and my daughter-in-law are expecting their first child in April, so now that I know the score, I think it's time I go into detail about the side effects of radiation, specifically no young children or pregnant women on my lap for at least six months after the start of treatment.

Goodbye, lap dancing; hello, balls that glow in the dark.

The front area near the bar is jammed with locals reading the papers, drinking, chatting; so young, so vibrant, so hip and so individual, even though all are wearing black. We go directly to the back and are shown a seat in the rear dining area. Lucky Strike is a favorite with visiting celebs, who stay at nearby hotels like the Soho Grand, a fact I'm oblivious to even after coming here for years. It's only after I notice all the tourists constantly eyeing the patrons while checking their tour books that I make the connection. I come for the food, which is first rate; no surprise there when you know it's owned by the people who run Balthazar and Pastis, two famous top-drawer, but more expensive, eateries.

I order a red wine, Nick his usual Jack and Coke. I opt for eggs benedict, Nick a burger and fries. I give him the scoop, trying to make light of the radiation. I want to make sure he understands that first and foremost I'm concerned for my grandson.

"You know you get more rads from getting your teeth X-rayed, but to be on the safe side, I don't think I'll hold Asher in the hospital."

"What makes you think we would let you hold your grandson, even if you weren't glowing in the dark?"

Nick laughs.

"Hey, I only dropped you once, and that was after mom and I brought you home from the hospital."

"I thought you wanted to throw me down the incinerator?"

"That, too."

We both get a kick out of that.

Over lunch we drop the cancer stuff, and talk about his work as a commercials director and the indie film he's trying to get made. It's a real thrill to watch your children pursue their dreams and to share the ups and downs of the journey. How about when they ask for you advice? *Heaven.* If happiness can kill cancer, I'm cured.

We finish our meal and head back uptown. No snow, but it's raining heavily. For my last birthday, Nick and Gil chipped in to pay for the film-to-digital transfer of two student films I directed in the mid-Sixties, and today Nick wants to come back to my place and watch them with me. It may be cold and rainy, but I'm walking in sunshine.

Separated by generations, taste, and technology, I'm afraid my films will fall flat and seem amateurish to my filmmaker son, but thankfully that doesn't happen. Nick especially appreciates my cutting to the beat of the music, now commonplace, but back in the mid-Sixties rare; and still cannot believe I landed (for free!) not only The Loving Spoonfuls but also The Beatles, the first soundtrack appearance for either band.

There are on-camera shots of me doing interviews, and Nick comments on how my voice sounds different from what it is now. I'm looking at my face and I realize my reaction to the younger me has profoundly changed. Before cancer it was just *same old, same old,* with perhaps a slight nod to a thinner waist, a less wrinkled forehead. Today, it's only a matter of walnuts. Is that how I'm going to mark my life—BBW and ABW?

Nick laughs when he sees me with a cigarette, even taking a draw during an interview. If I could draw back that draw, and all the others, would I be cancer free? Nick can't believe how I accomplished such precise editing on a movieola, equipment cumbersome and downright Stone Age compared to the digital revolution that has taken the movie industry by storm. I'm eager to recount the agony of that experience. Once more I'm distracted, and happily so.

As we say our goodbyes, I give Nick a DVD copy of the films, and we hug. The embrace is especially long and hard, but not too long and not too hard. I don't want to make it seem like it's the last hug we'll ever have.

Round 12

I'm up at 3:30 a.m., trying to exorcise my brain of images of things that can go wrong—for instance an allergic reaction to the iodine IV they inject for the CT, that can lead to shock and "Aw, shucks, he's dead." Then there's the possibility my body doesn't discharge the radioactive material they also inject for the whole-body bone scan, which at best turns you into a glow stick, and at worst, a suspected terrorist headed for rendition. I begin to meditate and try to empty my mind of these best-case/worst-case scenarios. I need to relax and fall back to sleep.

The next thing I know the phone's ringing. It's Helen. It's 6:14 a.m. She always gets up at this time, and last night when she called to wish me well, suggested she be my wake-up call. I quickly turn off my alarm, set to ring now.

"Yes—I slept fine. Yes—I'm up and ready to go—and yes—I'll call you to let you know how it went."

I'm in the bathroom brushing my teeth, when I realize perhaps it's not a feeling of calm but *fear* I'm experiencing. My body's shut down. I'm in a state of shock. Whatever it is, I don't have time for self-analysis. I'm running late and have to get to the hospital. The two procedures are carefully choreographed, and making sure I get to where I'm going when I'm supposed to have been on my mind since first receiving the instructions from Dr. Berman that I have to follow up with phone calls to NYU this morning so they can confirm the appointments. NYU repeats Dr. Berman's instructions and makes sure I know how to get to the hospital and to the exact areas (in two separate but connecting wings) where the tests are conducted. NYU assures me they schedule this tandem all the time, but I obsess about screwing up anyway. (Anything to avoid the real worry, and I'll be there.)

I go through the main entrance to the Tisch Building, NYU Medical Center, and follow the signs to the A Elevator that will take me to the Nuclear Medicine area. The windowed lobby, with light seemingly streaming in from every direction, is immense and architecturally very impressive. Hold it, is this a TV set or a real hospital? I expect to see a limping Gregory House approaching; instead it's a lime-faced stick figure in a wheelchair. I'm shocked by his condition. From looking just at his face, he can't be more than fifty, yet this cadaver seems twice that. Cancer—got to be. Am I looking at the future me? Is that why I smile—why he smiles back?

I follow the wrong signs (not everyone knows their alphabet) and have to backtrack until I correctly locate the A Bank and take the A Elevator to the second floor. The image of Future Me continues to be a distraction (lime is not a good color for me). There's a reception area right off the elevator, and without lifting his head from his newspaper, the fellow behind the desk directs me to go to my left, and then take another left and head down the corridor to the main reception area.

I pass three older gentlemen in hospital gowns and street shoes, sitting in chairs, reading newspapers, IVs attached to their arms, calm as can be. So, *this* is how they turn zombies into vampires.

I introduce myself to a woman at the reception desk, and after a momentary delay, my records are located and I'm told to fill out a consent form. The first section is simple, but when I reach the part listing possible complications, I quickly skip to the bottom, sign, and return the form. *Seen one end-of-life scenario, seen 'em all.*

I'm instructed to return to the first reception desk. The fellow working the desk is wearing a colorful shirt, and I'm thinking about telling him how great-looking the design is, but I sense he wants me out of the way so he can get back to his *Daily News,* so I figure I'll save my sucking up for someone who cares. He hands me a form, tells me to read it, sign it, take a seat, and when called, give the form to the technician. I take a seat in a row of chairs all facing a door that has "Vascular Medicine" tacked to it in bright red letters.

A buxom, mid-thirties lovely in a white lab coat passes by several times, and I smile at her in an attempt to reduce my tension and to get back on my game. She gives me the eye, but doesn't return my smile. Why should she? Either I have cancer and die, turn into a glow stick, end up in a dungeon with other radiological terrorists, or all of the above. It's hot as hell and I'm sweating, so I figure it's time to shed my body armor and take off my coat and my two layers of sweaters—a lot of good they would do, anyhow. I've got a couple of copies of *The New Yorker* Magazine and a great hardcover mystery by Ian Rankin called *Strip Jack.* I also have my iPod. Overkill? Too much stuff? Can anyone say, *insecurity*? I go for the *New Yorker*. There's an attractive woman in her late thirties sitting next to me, but I've lost that flirting feeling.

About ten minutes pass and the lady in white I've been eying appears, and with a distinct Eastern European accent halting calls out, "Rok—ess—pierre."

Well, perhaps this won't be so bad after all. I'm led into a tiny room with the ominous "Nuclear Medicine" signage, and after allowing me to gaze upon her full-figured beauty (in the most tasteful and surreptitious way), Lady Nuke gently removes the hospital form from my sweating hands. She scans the sheet, and to make sure nothing slipped my mind, asks if I'm allergic to anything, especially shellfish.

"No."

"Taking any medication?"

"No."

"Eaten anything in the last six hours?"

"No." I shake my head for emphasis.

Satisfied with my answers, she asks me to roll up my sleeves.

"I have rolling veins in this arm."

"Let me see." Lady Nuke begins to palpate the veins in both my arms, and I'm given to song.

"Left a good job in the city
Workin' for the man every night and day
And I never lost one minute of sleepin'
Worryin' bout the way things might have been
Big wheel keep on turnin'
Proud Mary keep on burnin'
Rollin', rollin', rollin' on the river
Rollin', rollin' on the river, Proud Mary keep on rollin'"

I wonder if looking at his bulging veins as I am looking at mine inspired John Fogerty to write this great tune, whose lyrics keep rolling through my brain.

"You're right. Your left arm is the good one."

"I'm going to guess Russian accent."

"No. I'm from Uzbekistan."

"Great country."

"You been?" She's smiling from ear to ear. I see a nuclear suck-up moment.

"No, but I have friends from there." This is a lie, but hey—when the suck-up gets tough, the tough get going. (I know, I'm taking liberties with another cheesy expression, but I'm under stress here.)

"Are you afraid of needles, and have you ever passed out during an injection?"

What a way to ruin a good suck-up.

"I don't like them, but I'm not afraid of them—as long as it doesn't hurt."

"That's good."

As she prepares to do her stuff, she tells me she's had big men faint on her and been forced to hold them upright while she finishes the procedure. I wonder if that's the reason. I fantasize about falling into her in just the right way so my head will rest between her breasts. Lady Nuke dabs my arm with alcohol, withdraws the syringe from an ominous-looking lead container, and sticks me. Seems like I've seen this in a movie, and I don't think they were singing "The Age of Aquarius" after it was over. . . .

Holy cow, as the great Rizuto used to say—it's painless.

"How do you feel?"

"Great."

"That's good."

I feel the warmth as the radioactive material flows into my lower body; the heat of the moment makes my penis hard. I fantasize this is all a porn flick, and in this scene, Lady Nuke feels my power, locks the door, pulls up her dress and let's the man with the glowing nuke get some nukee. I hear her Uzbek love cry as a thousands rads light up her love box. *I'm ready for my close-up, Mr. Oppenheimer.*

She's staring at me. *What? what?*

"Am I having a reaction? I don't feel my face swell, or my throat close." I easily clear my throat.

"Good—that's good. You should come back in three hours for the test."

"Oh, is that all? No problem, I've got to go and get my CT scan."

We make small talk as Lady Nuke removes the syringe, swabs the affected area with alcohol (probably from her Stoli stash), and generally prepares to get my radioactive ass out of there. I ask about the Russian restaurants out in Brighton Beach, and she tells me she and her husband eat in different one every Saturday night. I'm thinking of asking for a list, but she's busy writing on a card.

"You going to be radioactive until Monday, so keep this card on you."

Card? I don't need no stinkin' card.

Lady Nuke smiles and hands me the card. "You must show it to authorities at the airport."

Authorities? What—am I *The Spy Who Came in from the Cold*? Damn—why didn't you tell me!

"Put it in your wallet."

I take it and do as she orders. What if they shoot first and ask for the goddamn card later? I keep these questions to myself—the KGB has probably bugged the room. Lady Nuke opens the door and wishes me good luck. Okay, so she's not going to let me light up her love box, but how about a French kiss?

I follow the signs back to the main lobby and then to the G Elevators in the Schwartz Building. The Schwartz Building is a recent addition, and although the glass-and-steel structure is clean in design and coldly impersonal, I'm always reassured by the high-tech spaceship aura places like this give off.

May the Schwartz be with you!

The sign-in area reminds me of an airport check-in. I started the morning with two of Dr. Berman's handwritten entrance passes, and with one gone nuclear, I'm relieved to give up the other before I lose it. More hospital forms to fill out. So what's new?

The area behind me is all glass, and in front of me the people seem to be sleepwalking. I'm remembering Space Station 5, the way station in *2001: A Space Odyssey*, where the astronauts loll about before they make their connections. In front of me is the reception area, complete with telephones and copying machines. Behind the desk is a huge file room. There have to be four, maybe five attractive women energetically working the desk. Everyone is extremely polite, and when you catch their eye, they immediately smile. I'm sitting on a comfortable leather chair with padded arms, while my fellow radiological candidates, mostly women, do their sleepwalking thing, many muttering to themselves; upon closer examination I realize they're talking on their cells.

So I sit, stare, dream up stories about these women—a good time-waster and distraction that unfortunately never wanders into the wonderful world of sexual fantasy. Five, maybe ten minutes go by, and just when I'm thinking maybe I should be reading something, I'm called into an area off to my right.

I'm in a narrow, but cheerfully decorated, comfortable-looking room with five plush chairs on either side, each separated by a side table. I see the farthest seat on my right is empty so I go for it. I glance to my left and I spot three guys a couple of seats down from me, in their thirties, early forties, wearing regulation New York City Fire Department sweatshirts and ball caps. Right away I'm thinking 9/11—that I'm seeing first responders in the flesh, totally fucked up with toxins and on their way out; only they're shooting the breeze, joking like they don't have a care in the world, so maybe I'm wrong, maybe they're only here for a union checkup. Doesn't matter. Thinking about 9/11 reminds me of how lucky I am (see Lime Man). I'm overcome by a warming sensation. I close my eyes and say a prayer of thankfulness, then one to all those worse off then me; nothing like a good dose of radioisotopes to put you in the mood for some old-time religion. Next to me is an attractive middle-aged woman in a grey Chanel outfit with matching bag; across the aisle, a man in his fifties, tailored sports jacket, tasseled suede loafers; to his right a thirty-something looker. I'm thinking I should have worn my Armani.

To my right is a door. It's closed. I figure this is where I go. I don't hear any scary zapping, screams of fright, or nurses yelling, *Code blue*. This is a good thing. Tassel Loafers is sipping a milky-white liquid out of a clear plastic cup. He puts the plastic cup down on a side table. There are three or four empty bottles next to him. This is not good. The woman next to me on my right reaches down to the side table we both share, picks up an identical bottle, and fills her white plastic cup with the viscous liquid.

She smiles at me. "It doesn't taste too bad."

More smiles. I'm thinking the People's Temple, and we're all drinking Kool-Aid laced with cyanide.

"That's good," I say.

I want to say something clever, perhaps a reference to going down better with a sugar-coated doughnut, but when your stomach's churning at the speed of cheese, humor doesn't come easy.

There are empty cups and bottles all over the place. I see two wastepaper baskets. What—people figure they're going to die, so why keep things neat and clean? I'm thinking maybe I should clean up the area next to me, but I don't follow through and simply sit there like a stone. Within minutes a fireman exits the door on my right and another enters from the door I came in. I overhear them talking. The guys are in for a test. Union freebie, just like I thought, maybe part of a recently publicized 9/11 monitoring program? None of my fellow civilians look deathly ill, or terribly frightened, each, content to read and sip, sip and read. I can't believe I'm always the only Nosey Parker in the room—what's with that?

After five or so minutes, I'm called into a small office, where a young man in a white doctor's jacket has me fill out more hospital forms. He has less age to him than my sweater, so I'm having trouble taking him seriously when he lectures me on allergic reactions. He hands me the now-familiar white bottle. He instructs me to drink a full glass now, and the remainder in the next thirty minutes. The mixture has a banana flavor and isn't half bad. I return to the waiting area and pick up the *Daily News* that somebody left on top of a nearby table. I read about the latest Mafia bust. I start drinking. I play Nosey Parker. Nobody pays me the slightest attention. I should have worn my Armani.

Twenty minutes later I'm called into the changing area and told to get undressed except for my shoes and socks. Two healthy young things exit, and for the life of me I can't figure out what could possibly be wrong with such magnificent specimens, and I hold this thought until I come face to face with Mr. CT.

The room is cold, dimly lit, and it's small—dare I say, *intimate*? I think there was something in my Kool-Aid. The young man who gave me my bananarama introduces me to the CT Lady; she will administer the IV. I smile. She adjusts the table. I lie down. I stretch out. She places a pillow under my head. She smells nice.

"Just relax. Once I give you the IV, the test should take ten minutes."

"I've just come from Nuclear Medicine." I hold up my left arm to show her the Band-Aid. "I also have rolling veins in my right arm." I have been practicing this spiel since Lady Nuke sent me packing without so much as a Frenchy on my lippy-lips. (By the way, she could be a sister to this one.) I try to keep my voice calm. A calm voice means a calm body. Right? Right!

"I know. I've read your chart, Mr. Robespierre."

This is good. CT Lady palpitates the veins on the same arm, but down on my wrist.

"I'm going to give you one hundred CCs of nonionic intravenous contrast."

Like I know what she's talking about. I close my eyes. I think there's someone else lurking about, but I'm not about to look. Brace for the worse, hope for the best.

"I must not fear. Fear is the mind-killer. Fear is the little death that brings

total obliteration. I will face my fear. I will permit it to pass over me and through me. And when it has gone past I will turn the inner eye to see its path. Where the fear has gone there will be nothing. Only I will remain. . . ." Paul's in the house *with a gom jabbar.* The needle goes in without the slightest discomfort. I relax.

"You're from Uzbekistan, right?"

"How you know? You been?"

"Great country."

My eyes are still closed tightly, but that doesn't stop me from kissing up. CT Lady pats my shoulder. Oh, I'm good, but if you think I am going to open my eyes and follow up with a wink and a nod, you got the wrong guy.

I feel her taping the needle to my hand, then attaching the intravenous, and then I feel the iodine dye surging through my veins. No going back now. I am instructed to raise my arms and hold onto the sides of the giant, green, open-ended CT scan machine. No longer stiff as a stiff, I welcome the chance to come to life. I begin my slide into the doughnut's maw. Only my abdomen and pelvis are to be scanned. Am I imagining it, or is my lower body warming up as the intravenous fluid works its way down?

The next thing I know, it's over. A second *Holy cow*. I am The Little Scooter. It takes more time for the technician to insert and remove the IV than it does to have the CT scan. Oh, I forgot: As soon as the dye goes surging through my system, CT Lady asks if I'm experiencing any reaction, like my eyes or my throat closing. Does she not see the note on my chart that says, *DO NOT PUT IDEAS INTO THIS MAN'S HEAD: PATIENT IS NUTS?*

I open and close my eyes, take a few breaths and sense a slight tickle on the roof of my mouth. I message the area with my tongue. CT Lady acknowledges my discomfort.

"It's completely normal. You're good to go."

Go where—to fucking hell? *"Fear is the mind-killer . . . "*

While I'm getting dressed, I overhear a man and woman talking about how the city is trying to screw them out of their 9/11 health benefits. The woman is coughing nonstop, and when I come out into the waiting area, the first responders, both in their early thirties, look up at me and smile. I wish them well and they do the same. I leave. I'm really depressed now.

I have two hours to kill (bad choice of words, considering the circumstances) so I return to the main lobby of the Tisch Building, find a comfortable chair facing an atrium filled with plants and trees, and relax as best I can. I keep my eyes on the lush greenery, close them every so often in attempt at meditation, but I can't concentrate for longer than a few minutes. The best I can hope for is to focus on the garden. Occasionally, I can't help myself and I look around. Mistake. All I see is sadness. This is not the time to be a Nosey Parker.

I return to the Nuclear Medicine area and check in. Nuclear Lady is nowhere to be seen, so no flirting for me. Just as well, she may take it the wrong way and send her husband after me, someone I suspect is well over six feet and used to inflicting violence. *Can you say, KGB?* I attempt to read *Strip Jack,* but keep glancing over at the reception area. Anxiety really has a hold on me. *Smokey Robinson is in the house.*

> *"I don't like you*
> *but I love you*
> *Seems that I'm always thinking of you*
> *Though you treat me badly*
> *I love you madly*
> *You really got a hold on me (you really got a hold on me)*
> *You really got a hold on me (you really got a hold on me)*
> *Baby"*

After ten minutes or so, I can no longer get a hold on me, and go to the reception area and ask one of the Desk Ladies if she has any idea when I'm to be taken.

"I told them, and they know you're here."

"Okay, then . . . "

I return to my seat, but not before a young nurse wheels an incubator out into the corridor. I look away, but not fast enough. The image of the tiny newborn tethered to tubes fills me with a rush of sadness both for this innocent baby and the parents.

I sit and try to regain some emotional equilibrium. *I'll read my book.* But just as I scoop it out of my cargo bag, a male tech comes into the hallway and calls my name. This time I don't have to remove my clothing, just all metal objects, and open and fold back the zipper on my jeans. The small room is dark and cold, and totally dominated by another huge machine. Just as I did for my bone scan, I don't examine the room in any detail. I'm not interested in inspecting the weapons of mass destruction. *Just keep your head down, follow instructions and get the hell out of there.* Sure, some scary images will enter the neural pathways, but less is more (less to be recalled later and less to erase when the Freudian-Forget-the-Bad-Shit Degausser goes to work). Sounds good to me.

The tech asks if I need help getting on the table, but I show him I'm no invalid and hop right up. Alright, perhaps hop isn't exactly how I raise myself up, nevertheless, it's a nimble move; 8, 8.5, 8, the cards are raised high and I can see the smiles on the faces of the three Olympic judges.

The table is cold steel, hard and fit for a corpse. I feel its chill even with clothes on.

"There will be a series of scans taken. Two five-minute photos, followed by one lasting twenty minutes."

"Okay. Not a problem."

Obviously, the cold has numbed that part of my brain responsible for making rational responses.

"You will need to follow the breathing instructions that will come over the speakers embedded in the machine."

I do not respond.

"Did you hear me, Mr. Robespierre?"

"Oh—sorry—yes I heard you."

The first scan requires me to put my hands over my shoulders. I wait as the tech adjusts the table and the machine. Satisfied, he retreats to his walled-off area, makes some more minor adjustments. Here we go. My hands are still raised over my shoulders and I'm feeling an ache in both shoulders. I don't know how I can keep the position. Moving will screw up everything. I will myself to keep still by picturing the Death March scene from *Back to Bataan* when our soldiers force themselves to continue on, or else be shot as they fall. I see myself falling over the table and dying here on the cold floor.

When it's finally over, I complain about the pain.

"It's your rotator cuff."

Okay, it's my rotator cuff. So the tech understands. Is he going to do something about it?

"This will help."

Yes! He places a pillow behind my head, upon which I can rest my arms and take the pressure off my shoulders. This works like a charm. The last session is the twenty-minute scan and starts at my head and goes to my toes, unlike the first two that concentrate on my pelvic region. The machine is just a few inches from my nose.

"You might want to close your eyes. Some people don't like the feeling of the machine being so close to them. It makes them feel closed in—you know, claustrophobic."

"I can handle it."

"Okay then, here we go."

I'm not in an enclosed tube, so no problemo, unless—unless unseen walls will rise up around me and incase me in a mummy-like tomb. *"Three leaves a night to keep the heart beating—nine leaves to give him life . . ."* Can anyone say, *"George Zucco, show me your Tannis leaves!"?*

It's the proximity of the machine to my nose that's just the slightest bit unnerving. But no rush of anxiety, so I'm thinking, *I really can deal with this—this will really be okay.* I alternate between staring up at the tiny X located in the machine's housing and stretches where I close my eyes for ten, maybe fifteen seconds. I try to go longer, but I'm not successful. I'm through with the Bataan Death March, and while I flirt with images from *The Mummy* series, I'm now fixated on the machine hovering over my face, which reminds me of the underside of a spacecraft. I'm thinking of the opening of *Alien.* Poor Ripley, she has no idea what she'll have to deal within the next two hours, or for that matter in the two sequels. Neither do I. Better that way, I guess.

The X that marks the spot eventually moves down my body in such miniscule increments that I don't immediately realize it's outside my field of vision—and if I want to see it, I have to strain my eyes almost to the point of moving my head. Although there are times I feel like twitching, even imagining myself hopping off the table and saying *sayonara* to the tech, I remain rock solid and Chevy tough, and twenty minutes goes by quickly and without a hitch.

The tech tells me to wait while the doctors examine the film to make sure the machine got everything. What does that mean? Now—I'M WORRIED. What if pictures have to be retaken? Did the machine mess up, or did they find something? The room is completely empty. I want to cry out, but I know —"In space, no one can hear you scream." *They got that right, Ripley.*

A more positive person wouldn't entertain such thinking. *Well, let's go find one.* I lay absolutely still until I hear something. He's back. I turn my head. Ed McMahon's in the house: *"Here's Johnny!"*

"It looks good. Have a nice weekend."

That's it? No shaking of the hands? No gold statuette?

"Okay-dokey then."

I'm off the table and out into the corridor before they catch their mistake and haul my walnut back. At the elevators I spot two women from the reception area. Both have knock-out bodies; one especially is incredibly curvaceous in her skin-tight Spandex and funky gold-lamé jacket. They're on the way out to lunch, and while they wait for the elevator they banter back and forth with their supervisor. The sweetness of a woman's toes has never been a topic of discussion in my circles (where have I been, right?) so I'm naturally curious, or perhaps it's because I'm radioactive and I have spanking new sexual proclivities. The women's accents and the musicality of their voices make me think Caribbean. This causes me to long for Antigua or any of those island paradises. I'm also guessing their Caribbean supervisor, the one making the lascivious innuendos, is gay, and even though my two companions give as good as they get, I'm not sure they share her side of the bed.

We all get in the elevator, and as soon as the door closes, the two begin giggling about their men and how their supervisor is missing out on the fineness of something that sounds like *Rick*—only I can't be sure on account of their heavy accents or the isotopes in my ear. Now *I'm* giggling. I wish them both a great weekend and tell them not to break too many hearts. They want to know what floor I want. When I say I'm leaving the building, they tell me to follow them. We get off on B, then wander through a series of corridors, and suddenly we're out through the emergency entrance and onto the street. It is a wonderful journey filled with lyrical laughter, hair flying, provocative smiles, and boogying backsides. They know I'm lookin' and thrillin' when they throw me some very sexy bye-bye air kisses. I'm glowing the glow of the horny. Everything is back to normal. I decide to go home and write about it. I'll call it: *Share The Glow.* No, I have it—*Radiation: It's Been Berry Berry Good to Me.*

ROUND 13

LOOK at it this way—it could be Friday the 13th. Fortunately, I do no suffer from triskaidekaphobia. I decide to look up triskaidekaphobia in Wikipedia.

"Triskaidekaphobia (from Greek: tris=three, kai=and, deka=ten) is fear of the number thirteen; it is a superstition and related to a specific fear of Friday the 13th, called paraskevidekatriaphobia or friggatriskaidekaphobia.

There is a common myth that the earliest reference to thirteen being unlucky or evil is from the Babylonian translations of the Code of Hammurabi, i.e. the translation by Robert Francis Harper, containing the thirteenth article.

Some Christian traditions have it that at the Last Supper, Judas, the disciple who betrayed Jesus, was the thirteenth to sit at the table, and that for this reason thirteen is considered to carry a curse of sorts. However, the number thirteen is not uniformly bad in the Judeo-Christian tradition. For example, the thirteen attributes of God (also called the thirteen attributes of mercy) are enumerated in the Torah (Exodus 34: 6-7)."

I like this part, and almost go into Google to learn more, but why tempt fate? Let's just say today's Eric's Clean Scan Day. Right? Right! It's 7:30 a.m., and considering the circumstance, I slept well, getting up just once around 1:30 a.m. for a wiz.

Unfortunately, it takes an hour or so to fall back to la la land. Normally I'd blame it on the coffee I had with Steve at dinner last night, but that's not what keeps my eyeballs pinballing at the speed of light beneath my closed eyelids.

Thank goodness for Steve, always trying to keep my head above water, always trying to take my mind off my situation. Take for instance the day I told him I had cancer. His reply: "Can I have your car when you die?" To know someone would honor my memory like that is so touching. It gives me a sense of immortality, like having your children dance on your grave every year. When Steve saw me bang my head against the table, he told me he was only joking about the Caddy. Is he Mr. Sensitive Guy, or what?

You know what I think?—if you can't joke about death and dying, you've got no chance to make the most of a bad hand. Only when it comes one's own Kubler-Ross moment, not many of us make good entertainers. What to do, what to do? I say, amuse and abuse yourself in a world of smiles until *rigor* sets in.

Some of you may gravitate to clown school and paint yourself up to look like Clarabell. If you're in the Hunter S. Thompson camp of tomfoolery, the scene in *Fear and Loathing in Los Vegas* where Johnny and Benicio tear up Johnny's bedroom makes a good case for chemicals. The act of creation is a wondrous gift, so making things only recognizable in your weird world—whether from a kiln (careful not to blow yourself up) or ten thousand matchsticks (glued or otherwise fastened)—can induce unbridled hilarity. I have never been drawn to arts and crafts (no pun intended), but the act of reproducing thoughts by mashing out letters is a regular laugh riot.

Helen is calling to make sure I'm up. I tell her I'm in a state of meditative calmness. This is not my normal response to her wake-up calls. I'm usually a lot cleverer: "Hey, Darlene" (or whatever name pops into my head) "will you stop moaning and tell Helen if I'm 'up' or not." Ha—ha—ha.

I can sense she wants to ask me if [fill in the fantasy girl's name] is old enough to have Legos, but Helen's savvy enough to realize this isn't the day for the usual juvenile banter, part of her ritual when calling to wake me for one of our early morning TV appearances to promote our book.

Who knows when evil lurks on those medical scans? Eric does—and Helen knows I do, so maybe she's as surprised as I when I appear calm. It's true I meditate when I first awake, but is that really the reason? Have I actually learned to bend like the proverbial reed and not break in the face of an idiot wind?

In the not so distant past, all it took was a pimple on my ass to send me into cardiac arrest thinking, *Cancer, cancer, cancer*. Let me count the ways I drove myself nuts, and for what? Because I'm nuts.

Hold it! Wait just a moment, Masked Man! The history of Eric is: worry and nothing happens. Now, when I bend like a reed, cancer bends me out of shape. Coincidence? I think not. I can't take it. I shut my eyes.

Hysterical-Eric-in-the-woodshed-with-an-axe Migraine!

I look at the pictures I recently took of Lovely Blonde Nightingale. My head is on fire and my bed sheets soaked. Lovely Blonde Nightingale is my ministering apparition, and I find comfort in knowing she'll be with me this afternoon. I can feel the warmth of her hand holding mine.

"Eric," she'll say, "all the tests came back negative."

I'm out the door and on my way, and it's only when I turn onto 9th Street that I remember today is Helen's birthday. I'm ten minutes early, so I take a minute outside Dr. Berman's office to call. I usually like to sing my birthday greeting—though not all the way through, because I have a voice even a mother can't love. The arctic wind is blowing furiously from the direction of the Hudson River, so I turn my back around, manage to correctly punch in her number, then hold the phone to my mouth with my bare right hand before my fingers turn numb or the blast from the west freezes my lips shut; perhaps it's the wind tunnel acoustics, but I believe this is my best musical performance ever.

Later I'm sitting in the waiting room, and suddenly I'm remembering my first visit and I'm watching a robust, thirty-something guy standing just two feet away, calling his wife, telling her they've scheduled him for a CT at NYU, and I'm thinking this poor soul has cancer all over his body—and he's toast—and how if I had to have a CT I wouldn't call anyone—just take a long walk off a short pier.

Well, boyo, you didn't take that walk, did you?

Before I have a chance to think about taking that walk today, I hear my name called. No exam today—just a straight shot into Dr. Berman's office. Lovely Blonde Nightingale is nowhere to be seen, but I get reassuring thumbs up as Marlowe appears in an alcove at the far end of the hallway.

IMPRESSION: There is no evidence of abdominal or pelvic neoplasm.

I'm staring at the last line on page one of two of the ***Final Report*** CT ABD/PELVIS W/CONTRAST from NYU Imaging. Unfortunately, my brain isn't in full comprehension mode, and for good reason. I'm distracted by Dr. Berman, who is reaching across the desk and marking the *asm* in *neoplasm* with a spiral resembling an upside down six.

Then he's showing me another page, the ***Final Report*** TNO-5560 NM BONE SCAN WHOLE BODY, and marking the bottom with another upside down six, and near it he points to . . .

IMPRESSION: The scan is consistent with normal bone scan, other than mild degenerative changes in dental process in the maxilla. There is no scintigraphic evidence for osseous metastatic disease.

I want to leap across the desk, yank my savior up from his chair, and hug the air out of him. My second choice is to jump out of my chair, thrust my fist in the air, and, in my Marv Albert impersonation, scream "YES!" I do neither. My hands no longer threaten to break the chair arms and I'm also breathing better— the natural outcome of not holding your breath. I feel an incredible lightness of being, turn to the seat next to me, and wish it weren't empty.

He's writing—drawing—showing me—my schedule of treatment. One hormone shot—wait two weeks—external radiation for five weeks—wait two weeks—second and final hormone shot—wait two weeks—seed implantation.

"When do you want me to give you the hormone shot—today, or we could schedule it for next week?"

"Today."

Who said that? Am I nuts, or did I just grow a new pair? Dr. Berman nods.

The next thing I know I'm in one of his treatment rooms and he's giving me a choice of in the backside or in the stomach, where he says the soreness will be less painful. I choose the stomach. I still don't know what's gotten hold of me. Perhaps I'm still in a state of euphoria resulting from the scanning results. Sure, that might explain why I just said yes to the shot, but how could that explain why I'm also doing what I swear I never do—watch as Dr. Berman attaches the syringe to the ampoule and see a silver pellet in the ampoule instead of a liquid? Iron Man! I'm Iron Man, and I'm not afraid of anything anymore. (I just read synopsis of the film that's to be released this May, and it must have tapped into my psyche in a way only Bridey Murphy could identify with.) But that doesn't explain the silver pellet. *Wait a minute there, Masked Man!* Silver pellet—silver bullet! I get it! *Come to your fucking senses Eric, and remember your WEBMED! You're getting Lupron, the hormone commonly used for treating prostate cancer, and it comes in its own time-release capsule.*

Dr. Berman puts some topical anesthetic on the right side of my stomach, just above my groin area, and then he slowly inserted the needle. By now I'm looking away. So much for Iron Man.

"This is going to pinch a little. "

ROUND 14

TODAY I meet my oncologist at St. Vincent's Comprehensive Cancer Center (CCC). I'm still unable to shake this feeling of utter calmness. Sure, it may be a healthy reaction, only I'm not used to healthy reactions, so I'm betting it's just my way of numbing down the senses, which I recently learned is a symptom of depression. I have to stay away from Google!

I'm taking my digital camera, because I'm thinking of creating a blog called "Streets of New York," featuring interesting sights accompanied by a stream-of-consciousness commentary. Maybe "Ruminating Over the Ruin" is a better title, because there's so much homogenizing in the name of gentrification taking place it not only threatens to destroy the individuality of each neighborhood, but also when looked at in total, jeopardizes the entire city, because at its heart, it's our diversity that makes our city uniquely special. *Jane Jacobs is in the house.*

I put on a sweater and a pair of jeans, chosen for image, comfort, and for the fact they can be cheaply laundered and need not be expensively dry-cleaned. Something is wrong—I think maybe I should make a better impression. Why now? Why this doctor? A suit—do I want him to think I have a job important to the survival of man so he must save my skin, not fry it? A suit with a turtleneck, that's more the image when I go on TV to talk about my book or to a bookseller reading.

I switch to a blue pinstriped wool suit, black turtleneck, black loafers, and a full-length grey overcoat complete with cashmere scarf. Thinking of my book gives me an idea. Maybe I should bring a copy, autograph it, and present it to my oncologist as a gesture of good will and all that. Who am I kidding? Sucking up is what it is—but let's start off slowly and build up to the book when I really need the brownie points.

It's 9:00 a.m. on the button, and time for me to leave. I figure it'll take twenty to twenty-five minutes to walk to the radiation center. Registration is at 9:30 a.m. and the meeting with the oncologist is scheduled for 10:00 a.m. As soon as I get on the elevator I notice a change in the way my neighbors look at me. They seem to be more attentive and, dare I say, respectful? Talk about the unintended consequences of getting cancer.

It's brisk, but I'm dressed fine as I go cross-town, snapping off photos without a care in the world, when suddenly I hear my name being called. I turn around and see it's Mark G., a guy I worked with in advertising back in the Eighties. When I met him he was in his twenties, an assistant agency producer and a really good guy who did his job well, so I was happy when I ran across him in my neighborhood and learned we both lived in Peter Cooper Village—he with his parents in the apartment he grew up in, and me with my wife and kids. I eventually left Grey Advertising, he moved to his own place in the neighborhood, I got divorced and moved into Stuyvesant Town. Fast-forward to today—he's married, has a kid, and with both parents gone, he's now back in his PC apartment. Last summer we ran into each other in the Stuyvesant Oval. I'm shocked to hear he's recovering from a heart attack.

"How you doing?" I ask him.

"The cold air gets in my lungs and creates breathing problems."

"Why don't you wear a mask like I see the Chinese wear?"

"Maybe if we were in Beijing."

"What about your Lone Ranger mask? You still have that, don't you, or do you save that for your wife when you're playing 'Hi Ho Silver'?"

He laughs from the belly as if my riposte has tickled his stomach lining. "What's up with you? Where are you going?"

"To my oncologist—I've got prostate cancer."

"Oh, I'm sorry." He puts his arm around me.

"It's not that bad—my doctor hasn't asked for the money upfront."

We laugh. I'm unable to tickle my stomach lining, but I'm happy I haven't lost my gallows humor, even when the rope's around my neck.

"See you when I see you," I say.

"You don't look like Danny Ocean?"

"Just wait until I get some rads in me."

I hear his belly continue to dance as I turn the corner. I can't believe I so blithely admitted I have cancer. Is it because Mark told me about his heart attack? You show me yours and I'll show you mine? Maybe nonchalance makes it seem less important? I have no clue.

My plan to take photos isn't working. I'm taking too much time stopping and starting—stopping and starting. One last shot: two beautiful red brick townhouses, then I pocket my point-and-shoot and pick up the pace.

I'm crossing Eighth at 16th Street and see the Saint Vincent Hospital flag flying a quarter of the way down the block. I know my instructions tell me to go to the 15th Street entrance, the one where I met Ira, but I'm betting there are two entrances and I can enter on 15th. I look at my watch—8:50 a.m.—why chance going halfway up the block, only to find I'm wrong? Right? Right!

Whenever I'm in a hurry and close to my destination, I think everybody is headed in the same direction (to my movie or my restaurant), and I get anxious thinking I'm going to either wait on line or get turned away. Today, I realize how idiotic this behavior is—all these young healthy, bodies can't be decimated with cancer; even the people my age (rare in this neighborhood) don't appear to be sick, whatever that looks like. Sure enough, when I get to the entrance, its modern white façade faintly reminiscent of the Guggenheim, I'm the only one entering Saint Vincent's Comprehensive Cancer Center.

CANCER! There it is—right there in big, bold letters. Oh, the C word is always rattling round in my head; certainly it's been front and center on all the web info, doctor and hospital handouts, not to mention the copy of my biopsy results.

I don't know whether I'm suddenly feeling empowered, or maybe just facing the fact I have cancer, but I don't stop, hesitate, or allow others to pass so they don't see me enter; I walk swiftly up the stairs. The electric glass doors whoosh open.

The two front-desk guys, snappily dressed in matching blue blazers emblazoned with the hospital logo, greet me with broad smiles and rousing hellos.

"Hi, I'm Eric Robespierre, and this is my first visit. I believe I have to go to registration."

The older of the two, who with his pasty complexion looks like he could be a patient, scans a sheet of names. Naturally, I have to repeat mine twice and then spell it. Is there something the matter with the way I pronounce my name that leads them to think *Robespierre* is *Ginsberg* or *Du Pont*? Finally, he locates my name, and then much to my amazement, the younger one comes out from around the desk.

"Please follow me and I'll take you there."

My guide is young, built like a weightlifter, with muscles bulging out from under his tight-fitting jacket. It's a short walk to registration. Along the way hospital staff members smile and say good morning to me as if they really mean it. I can tell this because they look me in the eye and hold their smiles until I pass, smiles I readily return along with a nod and hello. Do I have a sign on me that reads "Smile, I'm A Newbie," or is this normal operating procedure? I think the latter, because these warm and fuzzy greetings go hand in hand with the physical environment, which, while being linear and modern, does have a caring, soothing effect, primarily brought upon by the careful selection of paintings and fluorescent-lighting system.

My guide hands me off to a gentleman in the registration office who motions me to sit down in front of his desk. He's also built like Hulk Hogan. Is this a cancer center or Gold's Gym? Ready with all my insurance cards, the registration process takes less than fifteen minutes and goes without a hitch. I'm given handouts and the ubiquitous indemnification wavers. Sign or die—so why bother to read it? It's that old masochistic me, looking for clues as to what can go wrong, because in theory, anyone I can't sue probably can kill me. Good news—I don't see any references to "Star Trek," so I assume the hospital's not going to employ Thalaron radiation, nor do I spot anything from Weapons of the Imperium. The last thing I want to see in my lifetime are Inferno Bolts—you know, the ones used in the Warhammer 40,000 universe to immolate targets and destroy them with superheated chemical fire. What a relief!

Armed with all my handouts—that include copies of everything I signed, plus more info on hospital procedures and prostate cancer—I'm personally led by the young registrar back out into the corridor and down the hall, but instead of making a left into the lobby, we continue straight down through the glass doors marked *Radiology Oncology*. I'm ushered into a small waiting room filled with patients, some in wheelchairs, some in hospital gowns, but most sitting in chairs and wearing street clothes. Several women are behind a long desk, sitting in front of their computers. All the women look up and smile. My guide introduces me; each stands and individually welcomes me.

"I'm here for a ten o'clock with Dr. Ng." (FYI: Ng is pronounced Ang for all of those over ten and behind the language learning curve.)

One of the women nods, checks her computer, makes a phone call, and then motions me to sit. "Mr. Robespierre, the doctor will be with you shortly."

I sit and immediately feel uncomfortable, because I'm not willing to appear nosy and meet anyone eye to eye; however, I need to scope out the scene. There are three rows of chairs and the man right across from me catches my eye and tells me that if I want to hang up my coat there's a closet right behind. I turn and see it's built into a floor-to-ceiling magazine rack stocked with a wide variety of magazines, and a coffee area.

"Thanks."

"You're welcome."

I walk over to the rack and spot the latest issues of *The New Yorker*, *Newsweek*, *SI*, *Cosmo*, and *Playboy* (*Playboy*!). Next to the rack is a giant coffee maker that looks so smartly designed I figure it must be German or Italian.

"Mr. Robespierre, please have some coffee, tea. There is also juice and some healthy snacks."

I turn. It's the receptionist closest to me.

"Thanks." My voice is but a whisper.

I've got my camera, iPod, and cell in my coat pocket, so I transfer everything to my suit jacket and hang up my overcoat. The man across from me is gulping down water and looks up and smiles at me. Can it be because my jacket pockets are bulging, an unforgivable fashion *faux pas*? Fashion Police—nah—not the way he's dressed, unless—unless he's undercover.

I don't know if I'm overcome with anxiety or just plain dumb, but I can't figure out how the damn coffee machine works. Fortunately, a doctor in a buttoned-up white coat joins me and shows me how it operates. It's really fantastic. All one has to do is grab a sealed cup of coffee from its dispensers (the flavor is up to you—tons to choose from), deposit it into the machine, place an empty cup under the spigot, turn on the machine, and in a matter of seconds your coffee is ready; and get this—the original cup has been miraculously deposited in an internal waste bin.

Naturally, I want to thank the doctor, but when I stare up at him (he's three inches taller)—I feel my body turn to gelatinous waves and I'm transported into HIS body. It happens so fast that all I see (with his eyes) is the top of my head and the mop of thinning grey-brown hair that lies there—I'm losing my fuckin' hair. Then *boom*—I'm back in my body—blowing coffee—feeling the vibration of my cell deep in my loins. Odd—I reach for the phone—it's not ringing.

I'm sitting down now, blinking, eyes aching, blowing on my coffee, cautiously eying the crowd for the man from the psych ward with the net and my straightjacket. A third of the patients are Chinese, each accompanied by a spouse or family member; in fact every patient is there with a caregiver—except me. There's an elderly Chinese couple (I think it's the wife who is undergoing treatment), and I'm not sure if they're waiting to go in or gathering strength before they leave. A frail, elderly woman with a heavy eastern European accent slowly walks in accompanied by a nurse, and from what I surmise, she's coming from one treatment and will have to go upstairs for another. She's complaining about the cold, and the nurse promises to bring her some blankets. The woman nods, takes a seat against the far wall, two rows across from me, picks up a phone, dials a number, and when connected, in a heavy accent I take to be German, describes the day's events.

I'm two sips into my coffee when a nurse comes out from the back and calls my name.

"Mr. Robespierre?"

The nurse is first-generation Chinese and is followed by a much older Chinese lady. "See you at 9:00 a.m. tomorrow, Mrs. Chan," she says to the lady. Mrs. Chan doesn't respond. The nurse says something in Chinese, and Mrs. Chan nods to the receptionist, heads to the coffee nook, grabs two tea bags, a little container of yogurt, and two health bars, and stuffs them into her purse.

"Mr. Robespierre?"

I forget Mrs. Chan. The nurse is looking around. I raise my hand and get up to greet her. She gives me a sweet smile and introduces herself. "I'm Nurse Laura. I assist Dr. Ng."

She's a tightly wrapped, no-nonsense professional. I bet she's a black belt and can kick my butt. I'm getting a "I'm going to meet the Zen master" feeling as I follow Nurse Laura through the labyrinthine corridors. We finally reach a series of treatment rooms and enter room number 2. Nurse Laura informs me that Dr. Ng will be in to see me soon, but first she has to take down some information. I hang up my coat (at the last minute I remove it from the hall closet and take it with me) and sit on the only chair available, while Nurse Laura grabs a stool located at the head of the examination table. I bet she can twist the legs off the stool and wrap them around my neck if she wants. She's got a thick folder on her lap, but before she opens it she wants to know if I've brought the info my urologist gave me to give to Dr. Ng.

I produce the envelope, remove the four sheets of paper, and she studies them. Satisfied, Nurse Laura opens the manila folder, tucks the four sheets up front, then, page by page, proceeds to ask question after question. I try to be as precise as I can be (I'm always anxious to show off my medical knowledge), but occasionally this tactic leads to convoluted answers; fortunately, Nurse Laura knows gibberish when she hears it and interrupts before it becomes too tortuous. After going through my file, Nurse Laura takes my vital signs.

"Dr. Ng will be right in to examine you and give you a sonogram."

She wants me to strip to my underwear and put on a hospital gown I will find in the closet where I hung my coat. I point to my stomach.

"Will it be on the outside or . . . "

"Internally."

There it is, then—the day's ruined. Nurse Laura senses my fear (all black belts have this ability) and lays on her best sympathetic smile.

"Will I get an anesthetic, like I did for the biopsy?"

"Oh no. This won't hurt at all, just a little bothersome."

Bothersome? A fly buzzing around your nose is bothersome.

"Don't worry, Mr. Robespierre, Dr. Ng is very gentle."

A hose job for a hose job—very good, Nurse Laura, very good.

"My biopsy didn't hurt."

"That's good." Nurse Laura gets up. She wants to leave, but I'm tighter than a vacuum-packed tin of Maxwell House; I need to run at the mouth and release the air. She hovers.

"Dr. Berman manually applied a topical anesthetic, then he shot some Lidocaine into the prostate. I didn't feel anything, just a little pinch."

Nurse Laura smiles and slips silently away before I can tell her about the twelve punches. (Ninjas can do that.)

I spend a minute examining the hospital gown. Common sense and experience tell me I have to put it on with the back exposed, but it doesn't seem to fit right (don't want the Fashion Police giving me a ticket), so I try it the other way, realize my error, quickly take it off, and do it the correct way. Just in time. The doctor walks in. *You don't want to show Savior Man you can't put on a hospital gown—maybe he won't think you're worth it? Right? Right!*

Ira hammers it into me that Dr. Ng is a really cool, young guy, that I'm going to like him, that he's really good at his job, which is handling the radiation part. When Ellyn first tells me about Ira's team it's Berman the urologist and Burson the oncologist, so it's only natural when Berman sets up the oncology appointment and mentions the unfamiliar Dr. Ng, I interrupt, say, "I want Burson." Something in Berman's attitude should tip me off, but it's only when I call to make my appointment with Burson that I learn from his secretary he's no longer taking patients, but devoting himself entirely to research.

I mention Ira's name, Ellyn's doctor friend, talk up Burson, but no amount of sucking up works. Complicating matters further, Dr. Burson is on vacation and won't be back for two months. The secretary then mentions Dr. Ng, informs me he's taking over (so he must be an oncologist), and goes on to effusively praise his work and his association with Dr. Burson. I'm in no position to argue, but guess what—Ng is also on vacay until March tenth. Before I can flip out totally, the secretary says she can give me a 10:00 a.m. appointment for that day. I quickly agree.

"Did Dr. Berman give you any information to bring to us?"

"Yes."

"Please fax that over."

"Okay."

She repeats the fax number twice in case I copy it down incorrectly the first time. (She must be psychic.)

"Please bring it with you as well."

"Okay."

"See you on March tenth, Mr. Robespierre. Am I pronouncing your name correctly?"

"Yes."

"Good. Have a nice day"

"You, too."

Fearing that a month's delay could be deadly, I have a fierce internal debate as to whether or not to call Dr. Berman. The debate lasts five seconds. (I'm probably exaggerating.) Dr. Berman's not in, so, as calmly as I can, I explain my situation to his receptionist. She doesn't think it will be a problem, but promises to pass along my concerns.

"What number can he reach you at?"

I give her my home and cell-phone numbers. I fax the sheets over to Saint Vincent's, and ten minutes later get a call from Dr. Berman's office telling me not to worry, the scheduling is fine.

For the last month, I haven't worried (*in denial, in denial!!!*) and the time away from doctors and hospitals was a welcomed relief (*in denial, in denial!!!*), but that's over, and here I'm am with my rear end exposed and vulnerable when

Dr. Ng walks in, brown as a berry, grinning like a Cheshire cat about to order a Mai Tai. I know the old saw that Chinese never look their age, but this guy is living proof the Fountain of Youth is on Mott Street—on the other hand, maybe it's blowback from radiation, and by the time I'm finished with my zaps, I'll look eighteen again.

"I'm Dr. Ng."

"I'm Eric Robespierre."

We shake.

"How was your vacation?" I ask him.

"Great, thanks."

"Where did you go?"

"Hawaii."

So—this is how it starts. How we segue into motorcycles from exotic women and tropical drinks escapes me, but we do, and if not for all-pervading fear of the tube going where no tube has ever gone before, the lurking inevitability of turning into a glow stick with not so glowing side effects, and last but not least, the omnipresent threat of bugger-me cells wanting to live free and making me die hard, my initial meeting with this intelligent, warm-hearted, and humorous Mr. Savior Man goes pretty well.

ROUND 15

ON Friday, I finally phone Dr. Berman and leave a message on his service to call me. For the last week or so I've been peeing like crazy, and just a few days ago it begins to burn when I urinate. The constant peeing is making life miserable. I can't plan any activity, let alone go to the store. Fortunately, there's a public facility on the Stuyvesant Town Oval, so I can take my hour's exercise walk around it, but a forty-minute bouncy bus ride up Third Avenue to see a movie is chancy, and taking the faster subway is even riskier, because even if you manage to get off in time, you still have to run up the stairs and find a bathroom.

I keep replaying the airplane scene in *The Savages* when the father (Philip Bosco of *Working Girl*-"Get your bony ass out of my office" fame) has to go to the bathroom, and as he makes his way down the aisle, his pants fall to his ankles, revealing his exposed diaper-covered backside. I'M NOT WEARING A DIAPER.

I will not let this problem destroy my life. I'm going to take a walk. It's about fifty, fifty-five degrees, and the kids playing in the various playgrounds are shirtless. I've got on a sweatshirt under a light jacket and I'm plugged into my iPod, listening to an audio recording of *Swann's Way* by Marcel Proust. The narrator takes me faraway from my own troubles, to his Aunt Léonie's home in Combray and her everyday household intrigues. Four times around the Oval is a mile, but I only make it a quarter of one turn before I head to the bathroom. The door is lightly ajar, and as soon as I enter I see an infant's changing table stacked with a half dozen or so diapers. Is this some kind of a sick joke? I quickly take care of business, once a joyous relief, now a painful nuisance. *My Hurtin' Pee—* is this the title of a country-and-western ditty, a dark ode to the fragility of the urinary tract, or just a notion preoccupying me to the point of exhaustion? And another thing—it's damn boring thinking about peeing twenty-four/seven, telling your friends (who really don't want to hear, but since you have cancer they must pretend they care) about the sleepless nights, the penis pain, the scrotal soreness or the force of your stream. *Yadda, yadda, yadda—boring, boring, boring!*

Dr. Berman doesn't return my Friday call, and I'm thinking, *Why did I wait all of Saturday and all of this morning before calling his service a second time? Don't I tell people, if someone doesn't call you back in a timely fashion, call again?* I'm terrific at giving advice, but when it comes down to it, I never take it myself. Always with the excuses.

So what is it this time? Obviously, these symptoms are the expected side effect of the Lupron; other explanations are too scary to contemplate.

Tough it out until September—don't show Dr. Berman you're a wuss. Right? Right!

I'm sitting in the Oval, basking in the sun, when I phone up his service for the second time.

"I don't see any messages from you, Mr. Robespierre, but I'll contact your doctor and he'll get right back. You're on your cell now, is that right?"

"Yes." I repeat my number. Something in her voice leads me to believe she will—that *he* will call back, so I head over to Walgreens pharmacy, figuring if Dr. Berman wants to give me a prescription, he'll have to phone it in, and since I don't have their number, I'll go over there and get their card. But I need to pee first. Back to the bathroom I go. Good news! Someone put the changing table in the upright position and closed it up. I'm hoping the place doesn't have a security camera. I don't want the boys in blue thinking I'm in here all the time because I'm a perv; not to worry, I've got Dr. Berman's card.

Drip, drip, drip—bodily fluids painfully dripping into porcelain oblivion. *Remember this morbid moment, Eric, and keep it close, so when I'm healthy again I won't take the wonders of a healthy body for granted, and maybe—just maybe—take time to say thank you to the Supreme Power. Thank you, thank you, thank you!* That's sounds good. I'm glad no one's in the bathroom. Then I think, *Cameras? Nah.*

I'm slowly making my way along the winding path toward First Avenue, past the basketball courts with the T-shirters playing with such happy abandon that I immediately feel envious and wish I could join them. The next thing that comes to me is not that I'm out of shape, could be their grandfather, haven't shot a basketball in twenty years—no, what comes flying into my head is that I'd probably pee in my pants halfway down the court.

I'm just about to enter the pharmacy when the phone rings and it's Dr. Berman. I tell him what's up. He tells me it's prostatitis and he wants to write me a prescription.

"Dr. Berman, I'm walking into the pharmacy as we speak, and if you can hold on a sec, I'll see if I can pass the phone directly to the pharmacist."

Dr. Berman doesn't think that will work, and of course, he's right. Too much hanky-panky; the pharmacy needs to make sure they're dealing with a real doctor. I get the number, tell Dr. Berman, and hang up, but not before I thank him for getting back to me so quickly. I'm relieved it's not the hormones; living with this nightmare until September would be just one notch under a sharp stick in the eye, and one above root canal on my list of Not in My Lifetime. I want to ask what the hell is prostatitis (I'm thinking biopsy blowback), but I let peace reign in providence and remain silent.

There's no one around, so I loiter by the counter. Oh, lucky me, within two minutes the phone rings. I ask the pharmacy assistant, Robert (my pal Simon's not around), if it's Dr. Berman, and this reedy, bored-faced, twenty-something nods his head. Boy—if the rest of us could save energy like him, there wouldn't be any global warming. I think I'll call him Robbie the Bored Robot. I sit and immediately feel the need to pee. I'm embarrassed, figure the bathroom's located somewhere in back, then I think, no—too many drugs laying around, so it has to be one out here in the store. I'll ask Robbie the Bored Robot (not to be confused with Farah the Bored Robot, who is re-shelving in slow-mo), but a woman momentarily distracts me, two seats to my left, emptying out the contents of her wallet onto her knees.

I'm about to warn her of the precariousness of this position when three credit cards and a pack of Marlboro Lights fall to the floor. I offer to help pick them up, but she nervously refuses. She probably thinks I'm going to pocket her valuables. Can't she see I have cancer, and cancer people are always on good behavior because they think this will save them from the Grim Reaper? I don't have to wait a few seconds before her lipstick, book of matches, and several business cards tumble off, but I'm not going to help because I suddenly get it— she doesn't want my help because she's not letting her illness get in the way of her life. Good for her!

Her attitude gives me the courage to ask Robert (I use his name, because I figure it's good to suck up) the location of the bathroom, but right away I know I have made a mistake, because the peculiar look he gives me can only mean he's never going to talk to me again or he's going to jump over the counter and punch me out. I smile. It's best to always smile, because then they think you're an idiot.

"Behind you and to the right."

He leaves out the idiot part, or maybe he whispers it to himself when I turn away. I walk a few steps and see tucked in the corner the employee locker room and next to it—a bathroom. I try the doorknob. It's locked. Whoa!

Robbie's grinning as he whispers, "The key's on the counter."

I look—but it's gone. I return to the bathroom door, turn the knob.

"Be right out." A woman's voice. "Be right out . . . "

"Okay."

I'm on my third hop (left to right, right to left) when the door opens. I rush in, take care of business, wash my sweaty face, return to the counter, get my meds (Robbie still smirking—thinks I've got an STD), hurry back to the bathroom (still empty), scoop up some tap water, pop the horse pill, funnel the water down and swallow—just the way I see it done by Andy Sipowicz on "NYPD Blue."

ROUND 16

WELL, I think it's about time I take another look at the patient information Connie at Saint Vincent's CCC gives me after I meet Dr. Ng, because no matter how many times I read it, it doesn't sink in. Well, that's not entirely true. I recall bits and pieces, tie them together in a fuzzy-wuzzy recital when anyone calls to wish me well today. The word I fall back on is *orientation.* I also recall that short of showing up, nothing is required (fasting, special diet, filling out your last will and testament).

I hope to heck I'm right, because this is an appointment a month in the making, and screwing it up would be an unforgivable act of self-destruction. I dig out the Patient Education pamphlet, and sure enough I'm right—only it's a "simulation." You say "simulation," I say "orientation"—maybe they are different, but I'm not getting my drawers in a roar or questioning my lackadaisical behavior, which borders on a major case of denial. The simulation will be at least two hours, and a slew of St. Vinny's best and the brightest will be involved in the procedure. I'm to get a CT scan, the results of which will be put into a computer and then digested by my radiation oncologist, a radiation therapist, a radiation physicist, and the CT technician who operates the CT scanner. This group of medical professionals (the term used by the patient-education pamphlet) will decide my course of treatment, and I do not want to tick them off by standing them up. So—how come I have trouble processing this information? Three reasons come to mind: denial, denial and denial.

Twelve noon on the button, and I'm out the front door. It's a brisk, beautifully sunny day, and once again, I'm giving myself an hour to get across town by foot. Naturally, I have my trusty iPod, but I'm no mood for more of my latest audio book, *Crime and Punishment*—although misery does love company, and at this moment, Raskolnikov's more in of a world of hurt than I, having just come out of his feverish delirium to hear his friend Razumikhin recount the fiendish murders of the pawnbroker and her sister which our protagonist has, himself, committed.

Like good ole Horace says, "Go West, young man," so I head through Stuyvesant Town in the direction of First Avenue. I share the path with people headed to work or exercise classes, nannies (and the rare stay-at-home mom) pushing strollers, accompanying youngsters to school. A twenty-something, dressed in a well-cut black suit, black shirt, no tie, and carrying a sleek black bag, is barking orders on his cell while texting someone else on his Blackberry. The cell is hidden somewhere in his pocket. The only clue he's actually on his phone instead of screaming at the squirrels is a thin, black wire snaking up from under his jacket to a lapel mike. His Armani-esque uniform reminds me of myself when I was in the ad game, only all black wasn't the hip look it is now, but more of an ode to Johnny Cash. We're walking stride for stride when I'm suddenly overcome by a familiar, wavy gelatinous sensation. *Whoa! Look at this! Eric, shuffling along, a little bent over, belly bulging and hair bordering on the unkempt. Boy—do I look like shit . . .*

There's some guy making excuses into my ear, accusing another employee, calling him *asshole* this and *asshole* that. I've got a terrible headache, but my body feels strong and tight. We get to First Avenue and I haven't the slightest idea what to do next. I'm shivering. I blink—the wave overtakes me and I'm moving again—back into Eric One. Eric Two makes a left and mingles with the crowd heading toward 14th Street. I quickly cross First Ave. My headache's gone and so are the tight abs. I tighten my stomach muscles and throw my shoulders back. I'm feeling lightheaded and my armpits are soaked. I look at my watch: ten minutes since I left my house. I relax my stomach muscles and resume my normal slouching shuffle before cramps set in. Beth Israel Hospital is on my left, but I'm afraid to look up and attract attention; what goes around comes around . . .

I know you'll be glad to hear I arrived safely at the cancer center, and at that very moment a man, with two gorgeous young things on his arm, saunters by. The women, identically dressed in stylish black outfits and sexy high heels, smile at me. The man calls out my name. I take my eyes off the women. It's Marlowe. He tips the brim of his fedora. I give him a thumbs up. I'm surprised how much his voice sounds like mine.

Twenty minutes later I'm lying on the hard slab of the CT machine, obsessed with the image of a blue balloon, slowly expanding. *God, please—don't let it explode and make pee-pee all over the place.* I'm concerned I can't hold my water, because ten minutes ago, I drank four cups of the stuff, the prescribed amount to ensure a full-up organ will "fall out of harm's way," allowing the radiation beam to hit cells in my prostate and only my prostate. I'm in a hospital gown, but I'm allowed to keep my shorts and socks—not the lead body armor I'd like to be wearing, but it's better than going naked. Dr. Ng is talking me through the simulation procedure, telling me all about the treatments, how many, what side effects can be expected, information he already explains when we first met. I'm listening with half an ear, just like I did the first time. Does this mean it's a full ear now? I have to sign a few hospital forms. I lift my head up so I can scrawl my name on the appropriate line. This is where they slip you the Thalaron radiation.

"Mr. Zulu, give me full thrusters and get me the hell out of here!" Captain Kirk is in the house.

Dr. Ng leaves, and Matilde takes over. Matilde is my guide into the wonderful world of radiation. She finds me in the locker room, when thankfully, I've figured out how to get into my gown. Matilde doesn't look more than fifteen. I am now convinced the blowback from radiation is eternal youth. Matilde is a radiation therapist. Matilde is also gorgeous. *Cancer patients must not lust or they will not be healed. Right? Right!*

Gowned strangers hover—all eyes on me, and I'm getting that center-of-the-universe-aren't-I-the-rock-star-feeling. I'm back lying on my back, a pillow under my head, my arms folded. Behind me is the donut-shaped CT Machine. To my right, medical equipment—nothing that looks too threatening to the untrained, but paranoid mind. I'm going to have a CT scan, but first a mold will be created to support my back, pelvis, and thighs.

"It will ensure accurate positioning over the course of your radiation treatments," Matilde explains.

I wonder if Matilde will sign my cast. 'To my brave, brave Eric. With love—Matilde.' Maybe she'll even add her phone number. *Cancer patients who want to be cured cannot lust—cancer patients who want to be cured cannot lust . . .* Okay, I got it. I will be good. The mold is blue and paper-like, and they use a suction pump to form-fit it to my body. The sucking sound is low and lasts seconds, reminding me of a toilet plunger—and that reminds me of . . . you guessed it. I pray I can hold my water.

Next, I'm to be tattooed. One tiny dot on each lateral side, the other on top of my pelvis, mid-plane; coordinating targets for lasers to correctly place me on the table. This positioning further ensures when today's scan calculates (with pinpoint computer accuracy) the optimum angles for the radiation beam to seek and destroy my cancer cells (and only my cancer cells) that will be the exact placement for each of my ensuing twenty-five treatments. I know—why don't they just get Obi-Wan Kenobi with a light sword and go real hi-tech?

When the mold is being fitted, I imagine this is how bad boy Kharis feels when they bury him alive in those spooky, black-and-white *Mummy* movies of the Forties, so full of genuine atmosphere and Egyptian mysterioso that they make the current crop of computer-generated hokum laughably fake. I wonder—at the end of these treatments will I also need the ritual of inhaling burning Tannis leaves during a cycle of the full moon in order to be resurrected to my old healthy self?

George Zucco with a fez is in the house again!

"A CT scan of your pelvis will be taken while you are lying in the mold. The CT scan is used to create a computer-generated 3D image of your pelvic anatomy, including prostate gland, bladder, rectum, and pelvic bones."

Didn't I just hear this? "Okay."

They keep playing with the table, adjusting it and my body (by use of a sheet), and I don't have to do a thing. Where are the piña coladas?

The scan takes a couple of minutes, but it's no biggie. You see one scan machine, you see them all. Boy, do I have the stones today or what? Easy when I'm going tubeless; no needles or torture-chamber goodies, just the daily dose of the death ray.

Please—don't let me pee all over myself.

"Mr. Robespierre, we are now going to align and X-ray you with our simulator. The simulator's X-rays provide a picture of the tumor site, and help us determine how radiation will be directed to it. The beams of the simulator are positioned to deliver the appropriate dose of radiation to the prostate, while sparing the surrounding healthy tissues and structures. We then verify the beam's positioning with a procedure called fluoroscopy."

After the X-rays, the lovely Matilde marks the area just above the pelvis and on both lateral sides with some kind of needle.

"This may pinch a little."

I wince. When does a pinch feel like a pinprick, when . . .

"Did that hurt? I'm sorry."

"No—it was nothing."

. . . It's a FUCKING PINPRICK! I wince again. I can't wait to tell my kids I got tats like they do. Hey, I have cancer, I can exaggerate—I'm allowed.

I'm glad to say I don't see aliens in the laser beams—on the other hand, they could be microscopic, in my body right now, heading for Ship Lupron.

Friends or foe? Only time will tell.

ROUND 17

I have my wish—9:00 a.m. treatments. Get them over with early, have the rest of the day to get on with your life—that's what Ira did. In fact, after his 7:00 a.m. treatment, he drove two hours to his factory, then back at night, and not once during those five weeks did he suffer any of the side effects. I should be so lucky.

Werner, my oldest and dearest friend, insists he accompany me to my first treatment. Werner's a serious and much gifted artist (favorably compared to Rauschenberg, among others) currently living in Brevard, N.C., coincidently up here to land a gallery show. We agree to meet on the southeast corner of First and 15th Street. When we make plans, I stress the importance of being on time and keeping up the correct pace, and Werner not only lives up to his promise, but also distracts me with his running commentary on women and architecture. (Werner's also an architect who once worked for Philip Johnson.)

We get to Saint Vinny's CCC faster than I planned, so I suggest we walk around the block at a leisurely pace. This idea works so well that when we approach the entrance a second time, it's 8:45 a.m. on the dot. I casually glance across the street, but no Marlowe.

I wave at the two gatekeepers. "Good morning! I'm here for radiation."

They nod and wave me through. The waiting room is crowded. I walk over to Barbara, the receptionist, introduce myself in case she has forgotten me from when I came for my *orientation/simulation* (she hasn't), and exchange hellos. Connie approaches (she did my scheduling when I finished by *orientation/simulation*). Connie is with another woman, who I have never seen before.

"Hi, Eric. How are you today?"

"Great.

"Hi, Eric, I'm Elizabeth. I'm so glad to meet you."

"Glad to meet you, too."

Elizabeth's cute as the proverbial button, and one snazzy dresser, while Connie isn't one to sneeze at nor to be ignored when fantasizing about hot-looking women you have absolutely no chance in hell of getting a smile from unless you have cancer. And Barbara's angelic face makes you want to make the sign of the cross in gratitude—unless you want the Big Guy to smite you where you stand.

I listen as Barbara educates me as to the routine I'm to follow. Empty your bladder while she notifies Radiation—wait for signal to start drinking—tell her when finished— she calls Radiation—if on schedule, go into dressing room— get into hospital gown—go to area outside Radiation—wait until called—get treatment.

Right away, I can see the timing has to be perfect or I risk peeing too soon or too late (i.e. on the table). I didn't have trouble during the simulation, except afterwards I did have to make three emergency pit stops (thank you, Starbucks) before I got home.

Werner takes a seat and starts reading a magazine. I hang up my coat, keep my cargo bag with me, but tell him to look after it when I go in. Every time Barbara's phone rings I think it's H_2O time, but it's only after the fifth call that I hear, "Mr. Robespierre, you may drink your water."

I get up and nod. "Please call me, Eric."

"All right, I will."

Barbara gives me another one of her great big smiles. How can I be getting goose bumps from all these warm and fuzzies? I want to wrap myself up in them, have them protect me from the death ray. *Oh, stop that! It's not a death ray—it's a life ray.*

I go to the food alcove, grab a paper cup from the dispenser, flip the blue lever on the fancy coffee machine, and fill my cup. I drink the cold (but not too cold) water right there, in two long gulps, then refill. It never occurs to me to sit down and drink my four cups in a more comfortable manner as I see others do. I'm too wound up, coiled up like a corkscrew digging its way into the hospital floor, water rushing around the grooves until it pours into the hole I'm creating.

While I drink, I casually scan the room. I try to avoid eye contact, but eye contact is not going to be a problem. Everyone is totally preoccupied. I can spot the prostate patients—they're the ones drinking or with cups next to them, and like my first visit, there's a large number of first-generation Chinese men and women. None of the men are drinking. I'm wondering what kind of cancers these folks have. I spot a Caucasian woman in the back. I'm sure she's wearing a wig. I quickly turn away from her.

As waiting rooms go, I can't help thinking this one is pretty nice; everything is modern in design, giving the room a cheery, clean, and comfortable appearance, and it looks so new, as if built yesterday. There's even a computer and I can see someone is on the Internet, scrolling through a news website. The Upper East Side Penis Pullers should take a page out of these guys' design book.

I'm again pleased how easy it is to drink four cups without becoming full or gagging.

"Okay, I finished."

Barbara looks up, smiles. "I'll see if they're ready." She dials. "Are you ready for Mr. Robespierre?" She nods, smiles up at me.

"You know how to get to the changing area and radiation?" asks Elizabeth.

I turn to Elizabeth. "Yes. Connie gave me the tour."

"Put your clothes in a locker and then go into waiting room."

"Okay. Thank you, Elizabeth."

"You're welcome, Eric."

"Werner—I'm going in now. I should be out in about ten minutes—at least that's what they tell me."

Werner stands. He's about six-one and at this moment seems to tower over me. I wish I could be sending him to get zapped, he looks like he can take it better.

"Good luck, Eric."

"Thanks."

I head off to the changing area. There are three changing stalls (all empty) and two banks of four lockers each (only one free). I take the key, go into the far left stall, and close the door before I remember I didn't grab a gown. I go back and grab one from the open cabinet marked *Clean Gowns*. If the sign were any bigger it would bite me. *I'm not nervous—noooo.*

It's really tight in this stall, and I struggle to take my clothes off, nearly losing my balance, finally realizing I need to undress from a sitting position. I stick my possessions in the locker, close it up, take the key, and after a moment's hesitation come upon the brilliant idea of sticking it into my sock (my gown doesn't have any pockets). I must remember to ask the technician if this is a safe place. I know when you're having a CT scan you can't have anything metal on you, or else it'll get sucked up into the machine.

As I leave I pass a Chinese woman in her late sixties, maybe early seventies. I smile. She smiles. Her neck area is discolored, but otherwise she looks okay. Burn marks—well, here goes any thoughts of wearing my Speedo at the Olympic trials this summer.

The waiting room is small, but comfy. Simply framed paintings line the walls, some pictorial, others abstract. I find myself drawn into one landscape, its muted tones mesmerizing, its vibe lulling me to sleep. A small-boned Chinese woman sits across from me, reading a Chinese newspaper. I guess her to be around my age (give or take ten years). Over her hospital gown she wears a faded, blue wool cardigan sweater that she buttons up to her neck. She has on thin, grey socks over tiny feet that barely reach the floor. I'm fascinated by the way she can hold them motionless while she noisily turns the pages of her paper. There is no one else in the room. So—who's using the lockers?

The door to Radiation opens. A man, about forty-five, enters. He's tall and well-built, with a ruddy complexion and full head of red hair. I immediately stereotype him as cop or fireman. (Probably neither, but why ruin my runaway imagination?) He nods, I nod, then he disappears into the bathroom to my right. He doesn't look too bad. I hear the man in the bathroom give out with a sigh of relief. He just made it. Will I be able to hold my water? I'm starting to worry again.

A very attractive radiation therapist opens the door. (Doesn't anyone want to be a model anymore?) "Mrs. Lee," she says.

The Chinese woman puts down her paper, hops off the chair, and follows the therapist out of the room.

I can hear the man in the bathroom cough, flush. A man about my age enters and takes a seat across from me. He's wearing a hospital robe, but he's got on orange-tipped blue argyle socks, much snazzier than my white tubes. I bet he's going to work, or is he a retired type who continues to dress for the office even when there isn't one? He opens up a well-worn paperback and begins reading in a relaxed manner. I'm surprised. I never thought there'd be waiting time. Tomorrow I'll bring a book; no sense sitting, obsessing about rads turning cells into crispy critters.

The man in the bathroom exits, nods in my direction, and enters the locker room.

Waiting time—I'm hoping I don't have to pee. The door to Radiation opens; another Chinese patient, this one a male about forty, exits. The gentleman's neck is also discolored. His hospital gown hangs limply on his frail body. I imagine protruding ribs brushing up against the cotton fabric. He's walking slowly. He's not looking so good. I smile, nod, but he doesn't look at me or anyone else. He heads directly to the locker room.

A male therapist opens the door a moment later. "Mr. Robespierre?"

I stand. "That's me."

This guy seems to be in his thirties, confident, not overly friendly, and judging from his swarthy complexion, either Hispanic or Italian.

I try to take it all in as I follow him to the Death Ray Station. Now, if both temporal lobes were functioning, I could manage it, but the left is too busy dealing with the emotionality of my body bursting into flames. I try moving my head. To my right is a room with banks of cubicles on both walls, and if you go by the computer screens, I make out ten cubicles on both sides.

This is Houston—five minutes to take off.

The therapist leads me to a computer. I'm almost rubbing shoulders with a second therapist, that's how close the stations are.

"Mr. Robespierre, could you please tell me your birthday?"

"September thirtieth, nineteen forty-two."

I look at the screen. Ah, my Orientation Day Photo. "I don't look at all like Brad Pitt."

The therapist doesn't even twitch. *Jokes—I don't need no stinkin' jokes. Okay—if that's how you want to play it.* That must be my chart, under the photo that doesn't look like anyone but a frightened old guy about to have his innards orientated.

The therapist is talking. "Come this way."

I'm thinking of mimicking his walk, only he's not Igor, I'm not Dr. Frankenstein—oops, I mean Fronkensteen.

Facing me are two doors: Linear Accelerator 1 and Linear Accelerator 2. Room number one is half-opened, the other shut tight. *Dum-de-dum-dum.* CAUTION: HIGH RADIATION AREA. *Caution* is written in yellow against a red background. *High Radiation* is in red against a yellow background. *Caution* is written twice as large as *High Radiation*. Two tiny icons (that remind me of a face) flank *High Radiation*. I follow the therapist through the half-open door. The door is immense and at least a foot thick. On the inside of the door is a very, very big wheel.

"Big wheel keep on turnin'—proud Eric keep on burnin'..." CCR is in the house, and I'm in the suck.

The dimly lit room is much larger than I imagined, and cold as a tomb. To my right, dozens of blue, form-fitting molds hang from clothing racks, each resembling a human body if you have less than 20/20 vision or suffer from "CSI" overload. In the center of the room is The Boss—THE LINEAR ACCELERATOR 1.

"The machine is capable of almost anything, but I'll still put my trust in a healthy set of tonsils." You said it, Dr. McCoy.

There are two additional therapists to greet me, both females, and when I enter they go into their routine with choreographed precision that would make Bob Fosse proud. One of the women lowers the table. The other brings over my mold while the young man makes certain I'm comfortable by placing a pillow under my head. I make a show of getting up onto the moving table with the ease of a gymnast, but they hold me back and lower it to knee level; next time I have to move faster.

"I took off all my jewelry and I put my key in my sock, is that okay?"

"Yes. That's perfect."

Someone asks me to pull down my shorts so they can see the tattoo. I do it with a little too much bravado, and may reveal more of my pubic area than necessary. I'm going to show them!

One of the therapists points a miniature ray gun at the dots, while the other bends over to take a closer look; this is a raunchy bunch. I close my eyes. The therapists take a great deal of time moving my body into the right position. They tell me not to move, they will do all the work. They move me by pulling on the sheet. Hey—I could use the personal touch here, but I'm prepared for the hands-off approach, as this is how they maneuvered me during the Simulation: *the Simulation—the Simulation—the Inquisition—the Inquisition . . .*

A therapist moves the table using a handheld controller attached to the bed by a thick black cord that appears to pulsate in rhythm to the movement of my slab. The group takes several minutes fitting me with the mold, positioning the table and getting me comfortable. They can take all the time in the world. If they don't get the positioning right, Mr. Linear Accelerator 1 is going to accelerate my organs into dust particles. Right? Right!

A camera is mounted up on the wall to my left, I assume connecting me to the computer room, where highly skilled professionals peer intently at their respective screens, calibrating and recalibrating, checking and rechecking each and every calculation. Right? Right! Also mounted on the wall, pointing right smack dab down at me is a red light—a laser. I turn to my left, and sure enough, there's one on the far wall. I attempt to look to my right (I'm doing all this maneuvering without turning my head), but that laser is outside my peripheral vision. *Let's see what else is up there on the wall. . . .*

"Lie still, please."

The lights dim a notch. I hear whooshing as the door shuts. Locked, loaded and vacuum packed—and ALL BY MYSELF. They certainly got out of here like "the fog on little cat feet"—more like last exit out of Chernobyl. *Dum de dum-dum . . .* If it hadn't been for the door—ahh, yes the door— well my initial description didn't do this bad boy justice. Doors like this stand guard over vast gold deposits at Fort Knox or secure volatile materials at nuclear sites; James Bond is always blowing them up—only in this scenario it's the real deal, and I'm the one on the wrong side of the door.

I'm not feeling the love here, boyo—no siree bobcats.

"Mr. Robespierre, we're ready to begin."

The voice comes over the loudspeaker. I wonder if they can hear me. Of course they can. I hear the whirring first. I have to decide—do I keep my eyes open or do I shut them? Mr. Linear Accelerator 1 looks like a robot with a screen embedded in its tummy. Its circular head is attached to a long neck that curves forward and droops down so it's not looking you in the eye when you enter. Perhaps that's a good thing. Two stubby-like, square glass armatures are attached to either side—think upside down J's with arms that unfold into sections. The circular, glass-enclosed head resembles a giant eyeball, only the pupil is square not round.

My eyes are now shut. I'm hearing clicks and whirrs, whirrs and clicks, as Mr. Linear Accelerator 1 begins his painstakingly slow, counter-clockwise tour around my body, stopping every so often to zap me one—a sound that resembles more a buzz than the old fly-swatting zap. I try counting them, but I'm thrown off when I begin timing their duration, and quickly realize each buzz is different in length. I promptly learn these calculations are a wonderful distraction, because when I stop paying attention to them, my mind begins to project images of me bolting from the table—only I'm not quick enough.

Stick a fork in it—the kidneys are done!

I will myself to think positive thoughts. *I don't have to urinate. Check! I'm not in any pain or discomfort. Check! I'm not cold. Check! And—AND — I'm not afraid! Check!* I close my eyes and try to meditate, but my concentration is broken in less than thirty seconds. I look up at Mr. Linear Accelerator 1 and try to figure where the rads are coming from. The head is the obvious choice, but so are the arms, because when the machine stops they're whirring and clicking, clicking and whirring, so maybe it's not the buzz I should be worried about. Then there are the assorted electronics affixed to the two sets of tracks, one up on the wall facing me, the other on the ceiling over my head. *Forgetaboutit.*

The thing I fixate on, and the strangest part of the treatment, is that Mr. Linear Accelerator 1 actually circles underneath the table on its counter-clockwise journey, stopping somewhere beneath the metal table to zap me.

Ladies and gentlemen, imagine if you will, a laser beam going right through the metal table on its way to Mr. Robespierre's prostate. Welcome to the Bad Walnut Zone.

The machine slowly moves back into its original overhead position and comes to a smooth stop. I wait. *One one-hundred, two one-hundred . . .* I hear a whoosh of air as Door Monster slides open. I move my eyes (still without moving my head) and I'm surprised to see a therapist at my side.

"The fog on cat feet," I say out loud.

She smiles. A poetry fan, or just a reflex? She begins lowering the bed. "All over, Mr. Robespierre."

"Thanks."

I wait until she stops, then I gingerly get up.

"How do you feel?"

"Fine—I feel fine"

"Great. See you tomorrow."

"Yep, see you tomorrow."

Golly gee willikers—you betcha—"SEE YOU TOMORROW" . . . Can I be any lamer? *Eric—they're killing your cancer, not your sense of humor!*

I'm a little wobbly, but I quickly regain my equilibrium and walk carefully into the hallway. The therapists to my right are at their screens and don't look up. To my left is another bank of computers with more therapists, probably monitoring the patient getting zapped by Mr. Linear Accelerator 2, or maybe they're working for NASA, and they're launching an unmanned satellite.

Well, well a little humor. I smile. *Maybe this will work out, hey, Masked Man?*

I look around. I don't want people seeing my silly grin, thinking I'm off my rocker. No one gives me a second look. I need to go to the bathroom. I enter the radiation waiting room. Two men—one in his thirties, the other older than I am—are reading and don't look up. Good. I'm not sure any nod or smile won't cause me to spring a leak. The door to the bathroom is ajar. *Praise the Lord!* I don't think I could have made it to the one in the main waiting room. Weak stream, but no pain, no blood. I'm really not expecting anything this early. Week Two, that's when the side effects start showing up.

I return to the locker room. Only the middle cubicle is free. I grab my stuff and squeeze into the empty room. I've learned my lesson and change sitting down. I'm in a no-fly zone of emotions. I don't feel anything. I know I have prostate cancer. I know I'm shot up with hormones. I know today I got a dose of rads that could kill a flock of geese at a hundred yards (well, I don't really know that, but I imagine so). Am I in shock? Is that why I don't feel anything? Well, actually, I do feel something—I have to go to the bathroom again.

I meet Werner in the waiting room.

"How did it go?"

"Not a problem. I feel okay."

"Good."

Connie looks up at me. "Tomorrow at 9:00 a.m."

"See you then."

"Have a nice day, Eric."

"You, too, Connie—you, too."

It's a beautiful day, and we decide to go uptown to see the new *Times* building up on 40th and Eighth, so we'll simply catch the bus on 14th and Eighth. I'm okay walking the half a block to Eighth, ditto the first five minutes waiting for the bus, but then I'm feeling a little bladder pressure, and I'm debating whether or not to find a bathroom now, or wait until I get uptown. The bus rumbles up and I decide to chance it. Why I don't remember what happened after my Simulation experience (urgency stops at three different Starbucks) is a shocking mystery, however, in the next few hours I'm going to get the message, loud and crystal fucking clear—I'll come to realize for the next twenty-five weekday mornings how four little cups of water will rule my life.

ROUND 18

I'M amazed I'm feeling so fresh and alert, and equally astounded that my body has the ability to fall back asleep so quickly after my blue balloon sees fit to irritate the hell out of every connecting nerve tissue and propel me into the bathroom on the hour, every hour, from 9:00 p.m. on, when I finally give up trying to understand The God Theory and fall off—so we're talking ten hours and ten potty trips (okay, cut that in half—in my present state of blue-balloon agitation, I tend to exaggerate).

I know, I know, I should fill the prescription for Flomax, and I swear I will today. Last night—hell, for the last week—I have been lucky, but who knows when my luck will finally run out and I can't get back to sleep; then where will I be? I know exactly, I'll be sapped out and a basket case for the next twenty-four hours, which is how my cancer cells must feel after being zapped by Mr. Linear Accelerator 1. Good riddance to bad rubbish, I say. Damn, I feel like telling my therapist to give those buggers a double zapping. I'm staring out the window of a bus and my mind's wandering to places only nut jobs go. Why am I on the bus and not walking over to St Vinny's? Because it's pouring rain, fool! *Jesus H. Christ on a Popsicle stick—get with the program and focus.*

Focus on the street. 14th Street, along with 23rd, 34th, and 42nd is one of the busiest through streets in Manhattan—dotted with restaurants, coffee shops, and those wonderful Starbuckses, a place I've continually put down for their homogenizing effects, however, THEY GOT BATHROOMS!

I decide no camera, but I have my iPod. I'm now of the opinion that music soothes the savaged urethra. I'm giving myself the same hour I take when I walk, because traffic in this town is predictable (always bad, and when it rains only worse), but today there are no tie-ups and I'm at Saint Vincent's in record time.

As I enter I spot Bank Lady in front of me, exchanging waves with the Lobby Guys. Bank Lady is a fellow patient, a lovely, healthy-looking lady in her forties. I first took notice of her last Tuesday, and after realizing we were both on the same schedule, talked to her on Friday.

"Morning!"

"Morning!"

"Morning!"

I wave, and Lobby Guys wave back. Call me crazy, but I feel at home here.

I'm a few steps behind Bank Lady and catch up when she pauses to open the door to Radiation Oncology. We greet each other with a smile and a hello. I'm surprised there are only two people in the waiting room. I'm also shocked a woman I don't recognize has taken Barbara's spot at reception. Elizabeth is also missing in action. I don't see Connie, either. *Masked Man, I don't think we're in Rad Land anymore.* Bank Lady takes it all in stride, and after removing her hat and coat, fixes herself a cup of coffee. I cautiously approach Replacement Lady.

"Hi, I'm Eric Robespierre. Should I begin drinking?"

"Hi, Mr. Robespierre, how are you?" This woman has a thousand-watt smile and should definitely work for Con Ed.

"I'm fine. Where's Barbara?"

"Jury duty."

Two *ugh*s, two grimaces timed to perfection. I like this unknown lady.

"We're on time, but I'll call Radiation." I stand quietly while she dials. "Can Mr. Robespierre start drinking? Yes." She looks up at me and nods approvingly, her smile amping up: two thousand, three thousand, four thousand watts of radiating joy. Boy, I bet she could give Mr. Linear Accelerator 1 a run for the rads. "Yes—start drinking, Eric."

It's 8:45 a.m. I'm scheduled for 9:00 a.m. and I'm thinking, *Do I wait a few minutes. or follow instructions like a good patient, and if things run late, just pee and then drink another glass?*

I'm consumed by the biz of wiz, which I rationalize is a good thing—better to fixate on Ng's anatomical drawing of a bulging blue balloon than on the dark side of the walnut. I hit the head, take care of business, and start drinking. Last Wednesday, I decided the lockers were too small, so I'm hanging my overcoat in the waiting-room closet. Naturally, all the good stuff goes with me, jammed and stuffed in my jeans pockets, so I have to be careful not to crush anything when I take a seat across from Bank Lady. She's still sipping her coffee. I think she's wearing a wig, but I'm not sure; the last thing I want is for her to catch me staring at her hair. No Nosey Parkers here—except yours truly.

"Rotten weather, do you have to come far?" I ask.

"Hoboken."

"Not bad."

"I just take the Path. I'm used to it. I've worked all my life here. You?"

"I've got it easy. I live on Twentieth, over by the river."

"In Stuy Town?"

"How'd you know?"

"My husband grew up there."

What is this—normal conversation? Well—why shouldn't it be? No reason, no reason at all.

Elizabeth enters and says hello. Boy, she must be loaded—I've never seen her wear the same outfit twice.

"You look very nice," I tell her.

"Thank you, Eric. Have you had your water?"

"Yes."

She picks up the phone. "Why don't you change? They'll be ready for you in five."

I get up and glance over at Bank Lady. "Take it easy," I tell her.

"You, too."

"See you later, Mr. Robespierre," says Replacement Lady. There's that glow again. I would like to take this mini-sun home with me.

"See you when I see you," I reply. I am The Clooney George.

I enter the changing area, grab a white gown (no blue-and-white stripe today), and look for an empty locker. Only two are free, and I take the closest one. Looking around and seeing no one, I decide instead of changing in the cramped confines of the little cubicle I'll take everything off out here except my undershirt and my pants. Oh, hell—there's no one here, I'll take off my pants, too. I stow my stuff, close up the locker, and lock it. The key doesn't work. I try again. Nope. I check the cubicles, just in case—still don't see anyone.

I hurriedly put on gown, try the next open locker; key works—yank out stuff—cram it into new locker—close up—stick key in sock—leave. I feel the sweat pouring down my armpits, and when I walk into the little waiting room I don't sit, but head straight for the john and quickly towel off. I stare at myself in the mirror. I'm pale as a ghost. I take a few deep breaths, splash cold water on my face, dry off, and head back into the waiting room.

I sit. I must have stuck the key into my sock in a way that it's pressing against my flesh. I fix it. Yesterday, a therapist asked me where I put my key. I point to my sock. It only follows that during the treatment I have fantasies of keys, toasters, cars, and tanks melting into steaming puddles of ooze.

Bank Lady has come into the room, but before I can strike up another conversation, a therapist enters. "Mrs. Kent?" she says.

Bank Lady rises. I see a glowing green bar of Kryptonite lying under my radiation treatment table.

"Mr. Robespierre?"

I quickly get to my feet. The place is deserted. "Where's everyone?"

She shrugs. "I guess it's the weather."

Obviously, my closeness to the Kryptonite gives me great insight. Sure, I'm not comfortable with this new arrangement, but I'm not going to complain—screw the pooch—however, I am thrown off my game.

"Nine, forty-two, thirty—I mean, nine, thirty, forty-two," I spurt out before she even asks.

She looks at me, then my photo and birthday info. Now it's my turn to shrug. I pause before we enter treatment room one. I'm curious what the other room looks like (the Kryptonite is always greener on the other Linear Accelerator 1), but I keep my mouth shut and follow my therapist in, but not before I detect a slight movement—the tip of a fedora. Marlowe has entered the building.

I've noticed there's a stereo on the front shelf, so for the first time ask if she can put on some music.

"Sure."

There's a stack of CDs, but I don't want to waste her time going through them all. "Play anything, I don't care."

I make small talk while my therapist expertly helps me onto the table. I know the drill, so without her asking, I open my gown and pull down my drawers to expose the three tattoos. I'm getting that blue-balloon-filling-up feeling. This isn't good. Maybe she shouldn't be wasting her time with the CD player? She turns away. The music begins.

"I think I may have to go to the bathroom soon."

"I'll hurry."

That's the last thing I want to hear. Fear may be the mind-killer, but it's also hell on the bladder. Suddenly the pressure's gone.

"Oh, it's okay—take your time, I'm feeling fine now."

The door whooshes shut. Let the rads begin.

I don't recognize the first tune, but it's pleasant enough, and I feel my body relax until Mr. Linear Accelerator 1 starts to rotate; it's then I imagine the therapist running madly from screen to screen, cursing her MIA buddies as she frantically punches the various keyboards.

I calm myself. Not to worry, everything is already set in stone. Everyone will be just fine. The second song, one that sounds a bit country, is mesmerizing, and I try to catch a few of the lyrics, hoping that'll give me a clue to its title. I'm having trouble until I hear the refrain, *"Be with me tonight"*—there it is. The third cut is also catchy, but no matter how hard I concentrate, I get no lyric hint, and to add insult to injury, I've lost the key refrain from the last tune. Doesn't matter, "Time After Time" is now up, and *wham bang*, the memory bank is wiped because I'm trying to figure out if it's Cyndi/not Cyndi, or is she singing with someone else—then I'm seeing her ten years back at a Halloween fundraiser— then I'm thinking the zaps seem shorter—then I'm thinking no one's watching the monitors—then I'm thinking they got me confused with another patient.

I'm so busy being pissed that I'm being shorted on my zaps that I don't hear the *whoosh*, and it's only when I hear and feel the table being lowered that I know the treatment's over.

"Uh—I only counted six, not seven bursts," I say to the tech.

"Nope, there were seven."

"Uh—I was probably caught up in the music."

No reply. Time to suck up, so I tell her how much I like the tunes, ask her the titles (she has no idea); ask if I can borrow the CD until tomorrow.

"Yes, as long as the CD doesn't belong to a patient."

"Great. Uh—am I crazy, but were the zaps, I mean the length of each burst, shorter?" She turns, nods and hands me the CD. "Durations change, but you're always getting the full amount of radiation."

"I thought that was it." *Yeah—sure you did, Eric.*

The therapist scoops up my mold and goes to hang it on the rack with the others. I look down at the CD; no jewel case. I insanely think of asking her to get me one—*nope—go—get—skedaddle.*

Do I go to the bathroom or change first? I get into the waiting room and see some familiar faces—the masseuse, the nice lady with the grey hair (Judi) whose hubby (Felix) kisses her goodbye each morning—get distracted, head for the lockers— mistake, big mistake—hell with it—turn—rush past familiar faces— make a beeline for the open bathroom door. Joy *to the world! Joy to the world!*

I dress, head out into the main waiting area, and grab a few health bars.

"Do you know the time for tomorrow's treatment?" asks Elizabeth.

I nod toward Elizabeth. "Yep. Beautiful sweater, by the way."

"Thank you, Eric."

"Hi, Eric," says Connie.

"Hi, Connie."

"See you tomorrow, Eric."

I wave to Replacement Lady. "Thank you for your help this morning—that was very nice. You all are so nice."

"My pleasure." She turns to face Elizabeth and Connie. "I've been a patient here three times—these people are angels."

It's still raining, so I decide to grab the bus on the corner of 14th and Ninth. Got to hurry—got to get home. As I sprint across the avenue, I fear running will irritate my bladder. Can't help it. The bus is empty. I take a seat near the rear door. I'm going to have to get off—it's only a question of when. I'm tense.

"What a day to give up sniffing glue," I say to myself and smile.

Nobody can hear me, but I notice a guy on the street looking up at me. Not to worry, he'll think I'm on my cell. I don't pretend to know the psychology behind it, but the sound of running water in the bathroom sink always hastens a wiz, so as I look out the window I'm thinking, in my delicate condition, will the rain beating down outside do the same? *I'm going to get the damn Flomax—stop being such a pussy when it comes to taking the stuff and—AND—stop reading what people have to say about the side effects. Dr. B and Dr. N would not prescribe Flomax if they think it would hurt you. Right? Right!*

I don't get it—miraculously, there's no traffic. Maybe I will make it home, or should I get the Flomax and use the pharmacy john, or the one at Starbucks? Strange things are happening—still no urgency issues as I pass Starbucks, hit Walgreens, fall into lust over pharmacy aid Shirika (who fills my prescription on the spot), and finally enter the land of a thousand trees. I know the recent plantings in Stuyvesant Town are not for me alone, but when you have urgency issues you return to your more animal state, and as my blue balloon swells with every raindrop—*woof, woof.*

Deserted paths, buildings hidden by tall bushes, and trees, lots of trees—*woof, woof. I can make it—just keep taking deep breaths— asshole—schmuckolla— why didn't you stop at Starbucks?—because I'm a Marine—I'm tough—suck it up, tough guy—breathe—that's it, just a little bit more—almost there—almost there—keep talking—keep talking—can't talk and pee at the same time—can't talk and pee at the same time—almost there—just up these steps—that's it—look at the pretty trees—don't even think about lifting your leg, see all the cameras?—down these steps—that's it—that's it—just a little more—almost there—I can see the house—so what if you pee?—you're wearing a trench coat—besides it's raining—pants are already soaked—there's my building—oh, hell—someone's in front of me—my neighbor—the Vietnamese banker married to the French baker who's always bringing home loaves of freshly made bread and never offering me* bupkis—*nothing,* nada, rien—*no, she's going into the adjoining building—just looks like her—a little faster—open the door—to the right—in the direction of the handle—into the foyer—press the button—elevator here—elevator here—yes—into the elevator—jiggle around—keep talking—almost there—almost there—does the elevator camera record sound?—who the fuck cares?* I'm jumping up and down. *Stop—this may make it worse—eight—nine—almost there—open my coat—not my zipper, not for the camera— out the door—two locks—top—bottom—no time for shoes—track water—dirt onto wood floors—who cares?—into the bathroom—pulling down the zipper—the worst time—out—out, you goddamn water spout—Yes!—Yes!—YES!—GODDAMN IT, THIS IS FUCKING GREAT!*

ROUND 19

I'M completely thrown off when I run into Elizabeth on the corner of 15th and Eighth. Sure it's CCC territory, but it's the old fish-out-of-water scenario. Thank God my Trapper Dan GPS kicks in, and after rolling through the cast of "Boston Legal," I recognize the woman at the vending machine who deftly retrieves the latest free copy of *The Voice* before the plastic cover guillotines her hand.

"Hi, Elizabeth."

"Hi, Eric."

I remember that first morning I saw her talking with another attractive hospital worker, thinking how bizarre it would it be to get a chubby in a cancer treatment center; how the boys from Planet Lupron make that the impossible dream. As we walk toward the hospital, I'm fantasizing about the female therapists, their gentle hands positioning my near naked body each morning in the dimly lit radiation room (Connie and Hospital Administrator Jane also magically appear) and I wonder how I can flush those fucking aliens out of my system.

"Eric, can I treat you to a bagel?"

I look at my watch. "I'm already late, but that's so very nice of you. It's 8:45 a.m., and I'm usually there by 8:30 a.m., which gives me enough time to drink my water and maybe get in ahead of schedule."

In the lobby, the narrow benches are filled. Visitors and patients huddle together, eyes vacant and wet. More activity behind the glass walls leading to Chemotherapy. Is *anyone* healthy? I head to Radiation Oncology and spot Barbara at the front desk. We exchange greetings.

"Should I start drinking?"

"We're a little behind schedule, but I'll ask."

I hang up my coat.

"No—don't start yet," she says a moment later.

"Okay, I'll wait."

I take a seat across from a Hispanic woman and her elderly father. I see them every morning. She works somewhere in the hospital and we always exchange nods. Today, the old fellow joins the club and nods—actually he gives me a little grin. Here is a woman who knows the score as well as any doctor, so I'm wondering—is too much knowledge a downer when it's her dad who has the disease? I go with ignorance is bliss.

Everyone else is Chinese. I recognize all the faces, and after six days many recognize me and greet me with equal familiarity. When I was in the antiques business I worked with several young Chinese women, and to my amazement discovered that they got my shtick, and turned into some of my best audiences. Maybe I can try something out with one of the nurses, get my libido going? A bit about Confucius doing his first stand-up in front of his very stern mother and father might do it. Where do I start? *I got it! "Hear the one about the man with hand in pocket? He feel cocky all day. . . . How about man who fight with wife all day? Get no piece at night. . . ."* Hah, ha, ha . . . At least I'm entertaining myself.

ROUND 20

WHAT a gorgeous morning, with bright sunshine and temperatures in the high fifties reaching the mid-seventies by afternoon, accompanied by warm breezes blowing into the evening hours. Week three and I'm waiting for the other shoe to drop. Why? Except for some aching muscles (from yesterday's mile walk, my first in months), I'm pain free. This is a good thing—so why do I wait for the other shoe to drop? Look—I'm even in the tub, taking a long soak in hot water and Epsom salts that in the past gave my tender muscles immediate relief, and is my skin hypersensitive, feeling any side effects—burning, extreme tenderness? No!

This is a good thing—so why do I wait for the other shoe to drop? Okay—Mr. Stiffy is still Mr. Floppy, but I've set him straight (wrong choice of words), promising him that next week we'll take Viagra, sit down in front of X-rated videos, and self-serve till we scream. So why am I waiting for the other shoe to drop . . . ?

ROUND 21

I feel really good, despite last night's jumping-jack routine that has me lifting the lid every two or three hours. Flomax does what the name implies, and certainly makes peeing easier, but my blue balloon still plays Mr. Stingy with the urine and continues to dole out its liquid treasures by the squirt. Fortunately, yesterday's two-mile loop around the Oval does a job on me, so I have no trouble falling back asleep.

It's another perfect May morning. The spherical blaze rising slowly over the Brooklyn shoreline is again putting it to me: *Hey Ricky-Ticky—you think you glow? Just watch me turn your little bathroom into an oven—suck-er.*

I'm lying in the tub, letting Mr. Sunny Show-off join forces with the restorative powers of warm water and Epsom salts to work magic on my weary muscles and I'm thinking, *The boy is back.* I'm also excited about my writing, although I still don't have a title, and we all know how important a catchy/provocative title is to landing an agent and then attracting readers.

Suddenly, all hell breaks loose. I feel something greasy in my butt. Damn— Mr. Linear Accelerator 1's got my ass now! I consider doing nothing, then I force myself to look. The water's clear. I wait—look again—clear. I hear the music from *Jaws*—see Roy running madly across the beach toward the inlet where his son rides carefree on his tube, unaware of the danger below. I reach between my legs—clear. I hear the drums of war beating in my chest. The battle for my mind and body thunders on with the Army of Angst (street name: Doom and Gloom) pitted against the Forces of Happy Thoughts (street name: Smiley Boys). I'm not sure who's winning until I spot a red, stringy thingy floating in the water and the sunlight goes out of the room.

I stare at Gunk Guy, bobbing so carefree between my legs. *Don't touch it and it won't exist—yeah, right.* I try three or four times to scoop it up, but each time Slime Guy slips through my fingers until I manage to outsmart it by using my entire hand to pin it up against the tub, and then inch Blob Boy out of the water, up the porcelain and into my hand—only to see Glop Man disappear into thin air, without a trace of its slimy-self

Dum-de-dum-dum.

What would Hugh Laurie do? Damn—if only I had a blackboard, piece of chalk, and a stumped staff to harangue. *"You can think I'm wrong, but that's no reason to stop thinking. If he gets better, I'm right; if he dies, you're right."* House is in the house now!

Fast-forward to the last fifteen minutes. *Mucus discharge!* It's asses to the wall (clean as a whistle, thank you very much, Dr. H.).

I shower off, move into my shaving routine—a little dicey because Saturday I cut myself on the cheek, and yesterday, thinking it was healed, nicked it open again. I'm doing a masterful job of maneuvering razor around cut when I think maybe I should check the side of the tub. *"Beware of the Blob! It creeps, and leaps, and glides and slides across the floor."* Steve's in the house, and I only hope neighbors aren't flipping lids, signaling they want to come over for an autograph. I swear sound travels through bathroom plumbing like a megaphone, and when the guy below me gives out with today's morning sneeze, I jump out of my skin.

"I don't mind the wind, but the rain . . . "

I always loved that riposte, and I repeat the line twice more. I'm revving down—even smiling.

I'm out in the fresh air now, determined not to fixate on Mr. Discharge, but I do decide I'll casually mention Pond Scum when I see Dr. Ng for my regular Tuesday-morning checkup. Naturally, I will put on my best I'm-All-Right-Jack impersonation; no sense in having the good doctor meet the real Eric Robespierre. Right? Right!

I get off the bus on Eighth (still too muscle weary to walk). Opposite the stop is the entrance to the downtown A and C. I decide my MetroCard is dangerously low, figure it's time to add another twenty bills. I can also dump off money from two regular Metros onto my senior card (Old Fogey Fare is half-price). Token Booth Guy says it's a no-go, but he can consolidate the regular fare cards, then when I use it, show my senior ID and get a paper pass for two fares. Naturally, I'm doing my best bobblehead impersonation (perfected in doctor's offices), so Token Booth Guy has no clue I have no clue. He's a courteous, patient guy (the unmedicated haven't descended yet), so I don't get cheeky, and wait until I'm walking up the stairs to give out with . . . "It crawls.... It creeps.... It eats you alive!"

I'm back on the street, walking north on Eighth, when I spot a police car blocking the street at 16th and Eighth. I check my watch and figure I've got time for a road trip. I quicken my pace, and when I reach the cop car I'm happy to see—*major crime scene, major crime scene!* I know this how? Obviouso! Paper cups turned upside down, dotting the street in a figure 8 and, AND—spent shell casings!

"Who, who are you . . . ? " "CSI" is in the house.

Did I also mention the two smashed automobiles? The scene unfolds: two cars speeding down the street maneuvering for the lead—crash—drivers get out, guns blazing. *Road rage, my dear Watson—road rage.*

I spot TV Camera Guy leaving the scene, but all he knows (or wants to tell me) is there was a crash and a shooting. Duh! I overhear a group on a stoop saying they heard five shots, and there's a bullet hole in the windshield of the Beemer parked a few steps away; sure enough, I see it. I take out my trusty point and shoot, circle the parameter, and knock off a few pics. I'm nervous that a detective might grab me (six are huddled in the street eying everyone, especially those taking photos). But not to worry—I will play the old cancer card if they do, but of course they don't.

When I get to the CCC, Gossip Boy must immediately tell Barbara and Elizabeth. They're hungry for details, and before I know it, it's a real gabfest, and for a moment I forget where I am—only all this forgetting makes me lose count of my cups of water, leaving me only one alternative—add another.

Tuesday is not only checkup day with Dr. Ng, but also the day the therapists take a complete set of pictures (check progress, make sure everything is honky-dory).

"When is your birthday?" the therapist asks me.

"September thirtieth, nineteen-forty-two."

I follow the therapist into Linear Accelerator 1. The lights are still dimmed from the last patient, and ominous shadows fall on the body molds, making them appear like headless corpses. I naturally think of the Zevon song about the headless Thompson gunner. I know Warren was treated with radiation—is this where he got his inspiration?

"It's Tuesday, so it must be picture day." This is a cheery icebreaker, don't you think?

"We take pictures every day."

Oops. The therapist grabs my mold, and for a moment I think she's going to bop me with the thing. Well, I don't think it hurts to remind them. What if Mr. Linear Accelerator 1 is accelerating when he should be decelerating? It's my body, why can't I double-check things—make sure they're doing what they're supposed to be doing—and taking pictures on Tuesday is what they're supposed to be doing? Right? Right!

I'm laying on my back now, not a very good position to further my position.

"I know you take pictures everyday. But I don't mean *those* pictures, I mean—you know—the three-sixty-degree set."

The male therapist leans over. "I know."

"Good, because I dressed up for them." I giggle, but my little witticism gets me no response.

Shut your trap, Eric. Tick these folks off, distract them, and gone go my gonads.

The therapists do such an expert job of placing me on the table and manually lining me up, the table moves only a fraction after the computer checks my position and makes its final adjustments.

"Ahh—if it's okay, I would love to hear some music?"

"Sure." Someone turns on the CD player. "Okay?"

"Okay."

I recognize the voice—the tune—"You're the First, the Last, My Everything." Someone has a sense of irony. I lie back. Out of the corner of my eye I see the hall lights disappear as two tons of lead-line concrete slowly whooshes shut. Mr. Linear Accelerator 1 comes alive . . .

"You're the first, you're the last, my everything."

Taking pictures requires an extra ten, maybe fifteen more minutes, so I might as well close my eyes and try to relax with Barry. I imagine all the great sex this man is personally responsible for and I'm thinking, *Locked room—lights low— treatment table—discarded hospital uniforms—Barry White! Oh, that's hot!*

I open my eyes, and Mr. Linear Accelerator 1's round head is coming to a stop, just inches above my body. *You know, don't you?* I wait for his answer. His red light comes on and he buzzes. *I knew it! I fucking knew it!*

Okay, Eric, time to listen to "The Man with the Velvet Voice" and imagine you have a beautiful woman in your living room, stretched out seductively on your huge, plush couch. Let's put her in a flimsy, silk cocktail dress (hiked up to reveal the gorgeousness of her welcoming thighs, naturally), and let's add the golden glow of a fireplace, a glass of the bubbly (Cristal, naturally), and something provocative she does with her lips that signals she wants you more than life itself.

I'm having the time of my life when my nose begins to tickle. I pray I don't have to sneeze, which would cause me to move, cause the ray to zap an innocent bystander. No way—the machine must have a cut-off switch. *Oh, you think so, do you, Masked Man?* I slowly sniff the ticklish stuff up my Northwest Passage and then down into the waters of my Southern Territory. I don't sneeze like any normal person—I send out a deafening roar (three of them), just like my dad. The sound and the fury scare the bejesus out of anyone within a three-mile radius, and lead all to predict a fatal shock to my system. Prostate cancer and sneezes that cause heart attacks—those genetic gifts keep on coming, don't they? Oh screw it! I smile. I miss the guy terribly—wish he were alive to provide the unwavering love and support he showed me until the day he died.

Just to be safe, I pull up three more sniffles, swallow, say a silent *halleluiah* when the offending tickle tickles no more. I stare up at Mr. Linear Accelerator 1.

"My darling I, can't get enough of rads love, babe
Girl, I don't know, I don't know why
Can't get enough of your rads, babe
Oh, some things I can't get used to
No matter how I try
Just like the more you give, the more I want
And baby, that's no lie"

I always say, nothing beats a good Barry White channeling to make the radiation treatment radiate. *Whoosh!* Lights, action, get off the table.

"Are you Dr. Ng's patient?" a nurse asks me.

I hop off. "Yep."

"You're scheduled to see him right after this treatment. Do you know how to get to the nurses' station?"

"Through the waiting room, the door next to the bathroom?"

"Yes."

Instead of walking through the waiting room, I make a beeline for the bathroom—make it just in time. Another moment and I'll be swimming to Dr.

Ng; I'm drenched in sweat. I know the drill. *Off with de gown, splash de water, and towel off, mon.* This is ridiculous—they get rid of my cancer only to have me die of a heart attack.

I approach the nurse's station and there's Nurse Laura, clipboard in hand, shaking a finger at me.

"I've been looking for you. Have you been hiding from us?" There have been times Dr. Ng's nurse appears overworked and so preoccupied she loses a little luster off that great big smile of hers—but not today. "I called your name," she continues.

"I'm sorry. I was in the bathroom. I guess I didn't hear you."

She leads me to a scale and weighs me. I have an image of an eighteen-wheeler at an interstate weigh station.

"I'm up two pounds from last week. I just can't stop eating."

"That happens."

"But I'm losing my Brad Pitt body."

Tittering like a schoolgirl, Nurse Laura dutifully enters my weight. I can't keep my eyes off her perfectly puckered lips. This is no schoolgirl who suddenly captures my desire, but a professionally schooled concubine, and I better get out of here before she raises the red lantern to summon her master, who would find the trespasser and kick the kung fu outta my ass.

"You can get off now," I hear Nurse Laura say.

"Huh?" I wake up to reality. I hop off the scale. I follow Nurse Laura to an examining room. "I just have to exercise more," I admit.

"I walk every day for an hour."

"I bet you do." *And—I bet you're naked under your silk whatever-they-call it in Fifth-Century China.* My God, she is a vixen! Just look at her—floating on the expectation of giving her man pleasure that will make his toes curl, ecstasy that rosies up your cheeks, gives you that endorphin flush and oxytocin high—works for me!

There are three adjoining examining rooms and we enter the last one. I'm normally a middle-room guy, so I immediately become suspicious. As far as I can tell both rooms are identical. I relax. See—when they put you in rooms with scary instruments (syringes, oxygen masks, and canisters) that can mean only one thing—THEY ARE GOING TO USE IT ON YOU.

I sit on the only available chair and she sits up on a recliner. I'm in trouble.

The recliner has some weird-looking equipment attached to its side that I missed when I first entered. The equipment is familiar. *I have it!* It's the kind of stuff you see in a dentist's torture chamber so—unless the chair turns me upside down—I'm okay.

Nurse Laura opens my chart. "So, how are you doing, Eric?"

Oh, fine if you don't count the ten morning heart attacks before I get to a bathroom.

"Oh, just the normal urgency problems." I force a smile. "I'm really very lucky

"That's good. No rectal bleeding, trouble peeing?"

I casually mention the blob (naturally, I call it a discharge), but she doesn't appear too concerned, and only wants to make sure I'm taking my Flomax. I quickly realize my mistake—I didn't make it sound serious enough. Before I retell my story to Dr. Ng, I'll hum a few bars from *Jaws.*

Nurse Laura rises. "Dr. Ng will be right in."

What—no flirting with the cancer patients so they feel better? These Tuesday meetings are getting to be a drag. As Nurse Laura leaves I spot something on the floor. It's a magnifier on a headband. I don't even want to think about what it's used for. Do I pick it up or leave it there? I'm unable to think of anything else.

Thank goodness this idiocy is finally interrupted when I hear voices out in the hallway. Dr. Ng—and it sounds like he's talking to *GQ* Lou, a fellow prostate cancer patient I met in the locker room, whose demeanor made me think of Fernando's famous words. I whisper them to myself in my best Billy Crystal doing Fernando Lamas Spanish accent: "*It's better to look good than to feel good.*"

I hear Dr. Ng say something to Lou; then I hear Lou laughing. This is good for Lou. I smile. Words of encouragement from Dr. Ng, even if it's not exactly what Lou's looking for; then again, no doctor in the world can tell you how much longer you have to live. I can't hear exactly who is saying what to whom, but the laughter persists until the door opens, and in walks a smiling Dr. Ng.

He hoists himself up onto the recliner, opens my chart, and says hello.

"You look well. How was your weekend, Dr. Ng?"

"Nice, but I had to come in to the hospital on Saturday for meetings."

This guy's a saint. How lucky am I? I wrap my hospital gown tighter around me to warm myself from the sudden chill. "How was the ride in on your scooter?" I ask.

"Great." He looks surprised.

"I saw it when I came in, and then heard someone mention it was yours. How come you didn't ride your big bike?"

"I switch off."

"What is it again—I can't remember?"

"Ducati."

"Ducati—that's it—and it's red, right?"

"How did you know?" He's grinning from ear to ear.

"It's the sharpest color and you're a sharp-looking guy."

Before you say, *Ahh, there goes Eric brown-nosing the doctors again*, I have to say in my defense, when I'm overcome by feelings of well-being (i.e. I'M NOT GOING TO DIE!), I tend to get all mushy inside and gush compliments. In olden times I'd be the serf who prostrates himself in front of his master and kisses his feet when he's spared the axe. (By the by, these compliments are totally deserved—Dr. Ng *is* one cool dude.)

We talk some more about his motorcycle and I can see he's an avid biker, but I'm thinking, *How do I get to Mr. Blob? Let the conversation play out—don't let on you care more about your* tush *than how easy it is to downshift on a Ducati.*

Sure enough, he wants to know how I'm doing, and I tell him that besides the peeing I got me a little "mucus discharge," figuring I can impress him with a little doc speak. Maybe now's a good time to tell him I had two years pre-med at NYU. Eh, screw that. I don't want him to know two Ds in organic chemistry nearly got me the boot.

What is he saying?

"Sounds normal, but I'll check you out in a moment."

He wants to know if I'm taking the Flomax.

"Yep. I only wake up every three hours, but there's no constriction or pain."

"No burning?"

"Nope."

I hate it when he talks about symptoms I don't have. Doesn't he know he's talking to Mr. Psycho Psychosis?

Come on, you're Marlowe-tough. Pull your fedora down and deal with it when you deal with it.

"Take Aleve. It will relax the muscles and stop you from peeing so frequently."

"Sounds good, I'll try it."

"Time for a butt check."

Damn—I was hoping he would forget. On with the latex gloves and up with the fingers, but no, it's only a little spread. All right then!

He closes my file, stands, but before he leaves I ask him how my pictures turned out.

"Which ones? We take pictures every day."

"Oh—you know, the total body three-sixties."

"Fine—they came out fine."

"What about the dead cancer cells, can you see them in the pictures?"

He stops. Maybe I should have, too.

"No, the only way you can see them is through a microscope."

"You mean from a biopsy?"

"Yes—but we're not going to do that. We never do biopsies. We check your PSA."

"So—if the PSA goes up that means you didn't kill all the cells?"

"No—the PSA score goes up because cancer cells too small to be picked up by present screening methods escaped the prostate before treatment began and now are large enough to be detected."

The light bulb goes off, and I finally get it! "That's why Dr. Berman gives me only an eighty-five percent chance of a full recovery. The remaining fifteen percent covers the possibility undetected cells may have gotten out."

Dr. Ng nods. He stands. "Friday, I'm going to bring in the Ducati so you can see it."

"Great—I'll keep my eyes open for it."

It's gush time again. I don't know how this guy does it. It must be his aura that just sends out feelings of well-being. I want to hug the guy. I want to tell everyone with prostate cancer IT WILL BE ALL RIGHT! Too bad the glow goes when Dr. Ng goes. I follow him out. I say hi to the three nurses at the nurses' station and head for the changing area, but open the wrong door and come face to face with an unfamiliar corridor. A radiation therapist immediately understands my predicament and points to the right one door.

"I still don't know where I'm going."

"That's okay—everybody gets lost around here."

I'm not focusing. It's those treacherous fifteen-percent fuckers; those deadly invisible cancer cells who long ago wiggled out of my prostate and are just waiting to show up in bones or someplace even more life threatening. It goes without saying, these sadistic little buggers won't seek and destroy until I'm dosed—seeded with enough rads to make the scene in *Raiders of the Lost Ark* (when the bad boys open the ark and get melted down like candle wax) pale in comparison.

I can't fixate on this horrible image beyond the changing area; so many pit stops, so little time, and, you know me—I can't obsess and pee at the same time.

ROUND 22

AS you would expect, the thing I'm most interested in when I get to the dermatologist is the location of the nearest bathroom. I'm pretty sure I'm watered out, but like the old trapper says, *"Keep on pissin' 'til the bladder's so dry it can set itself on fire."*

I've got this little pimple on the side of my nose that won't heal, and because I know this is one of the signs of skin cancer, I finally decide to have it checked out. I fill out the forms and for the first time have to fill in the space that deals with current illnesses. I write "prostate cancer." I look around the room. Nobody is watching. Here I am, confronting the fact that I have cancer, and no one gives a shit.

I return the form, hit the head, and come back into the waiting room. Every chair is filled, and for the first time, I notice how many gorgeous model-types are sitting across from me. Maybe five out of the eight people waiting look like they just stepped off the front page of *Vogue*. No wonder they don't give me the time of day. For the next hour, I watch in amazement as these out-of-this-world beauties vanish into a side area while the rest of us mere mortals wait, and wait, and wait some more, until we are eventually admitted to the treatment rooms located in the rear. I recall recently reading on a medical advocates' blog the reason for my wait. Apparently, the insured wait, while the cash customers cash in. *Who knows what evil lurks? The Shadow does . . .*

Dr. A is all business, and after giving me some ointment, tells me to come back in two weeks if it doesn't clear up, and he'll take a biopsy. I don't know what's in the ointment and if it's going to play nicely with the radiation or set my nose on fire—so I tell him I have prostate cancer. I've never seen him so interested. He wants to know how I found out, what my PSA score was and what treatment I chose.

When the appointment's done, I hit the lavatory one last tinkle time, and then I'm out the door. I can't shake the feeling the doc's really worried about *his* prostate.

Well, I can't be more upbeat than I am in his office. I'm happy they caught it in time. I'm happy it hasn't spread. I'm happy with the doctors and their treatment.

Hey Dr. Derma-tol-logist—catch the vibe. I'm just one happy guy . . .

ROUND 23

AFTER my treatment, Connie gives me a sheet of paper, instructs me to go and have my blood taken, a chest x-ray, then an EKG. Appointments for these pre-op procedures are made back in April, and must be scheduled for a day two weeks before my June surgery. If I don't keep these appointments, no seed implantation. But don't think I don't think about skipping out after this morning's zapping.

There are letters attached to each procedure, indicating exactly where on the floor I'm to go. Naturally I get lost (the simpler it is, the more simpleminded I get), so I have to return, get more specific directions from Connie without making out how dumb I am, then find my way to the door marked *D*. I can't believe I can't find it the first time. The center is really not that big, nor mazelike in its design. Everything is on one floor and laid out in the shape of a T, only the horizontal is many times longer than the vertical. The bottom of the T is the entrance. A few steps up the T and to the left is the entrance to the Breast Cancer Center. At the top of the T is the Chemotherapy area. Make a left at the top, and down the hall is Radiation Oncology. Make a right at the top of the T and you see a corridor lined with inviting waiting areas on the left, and offices, examination and treatment areas to the right. The first office is Registration, then territory that will soon be known to me.

Each area is marked with a letter of the alphabet, located above the entrance way and clearly visible, except to me. Bloodletting (D), my first destination, is the second letter down from Registration (which is marked with an E above its portal). Obviously, I miss these markings, because I'm suffering the effects of dopiness due to smart-cell radiation eradication (DSCRERAD for short, and pronounced the way it looks). I have to remember to ask Dr. Ng if he's got anything I can take for it.

I notice area J (for my EKG) is all the way down the hall, but where is B (Radiology), the place I'm to go for chest X-ray? *I'll cross that bridge when I get to it*, as William Holden must have muttered to Jack Hawkins in *The Bridge on The River Kwai* or maybe to Mickey Rooney in the *The Bridges at Toko-Ri*.

I go into D and hand the young man my bloodletting document, which he casually glances at until he dismissively waves it at me.

"Wait outside until I call you."

I'm momentarily flummoxed. Where was this guy when they were handing out the nice pills? Maybe he's a temp and missed his meds? There's only one way to deal with guys like this. If only I could glow—just in the ears, but enough to make people's hair stand up and begin to crackle, "Hey, Sparky, you want me to wait WHERE?" That would be truly RAD!

I find a comfortable seat in the waiting area, take in the watercolors on the highly polished walls, the plants that seem to be growing from out of the floor in gleaming silver pots, and my neighbors. The latter is a mistake. A couple I guess to be husband and wife sit next to me. Both look ill and so tragic. I immediately make up stories. He's been dying for over a year, but now she's been diagnosed with a fatal disease that will kill her in days. She's long-suffering and he's so stressed out he's on the verge of a heart attack.

I'm completely wrong. They stand as a woman in her thirties comes out of Bloodletting, clutching a ream of admittance forms—their daughter! She's the one who has cancer. They move away. Before I have a chance to get depressed, a hospital person catches my eye and, smiles.

"Hi, how are you today?" she says.

I can't help but smile as I return the greeting. It's a nonstop procession of good cheer as doctors, nurses, therapists, and technicians all take the time to show me they care. I don't want to leave.

I can't read or listen to my iPod. Too much is happening, and besides, I've got peeing on my mind. I can either go back to Radiation Oncology or try to find one here.

"Mr. Robespierre."

It's Sparky. I look up.

He continues. "Yes. I'm sorry—we do not have your name on our list."

"Connie told me to come here. Why don't you call her?"

"I don't know any Connie."

"Okay."

He hands me my paper, turns his back on me, and walks away. Remember the "I'll be back" scene from *Terminator*? Sure, I can say the words, but where's the assault weapon when you really need it? I slowly make my way back to Radiation. Oh well, at least I can use the bathroom.

Ten minutes later I'm back in Bloodletting, relieved the person sticking me isn't the one Connie just stuck it to. There must be six or more stations in this tiny, windowless room, each one decorated with filled racks of tubing and vials. People are rolling up or rolling down their sleeves in unison—like a well-choreographed Busby Berkeley dance routine. I'm impressed. These technicians are pros, and the exotic young lovely who takes me to her station is no exception. She reads my paper carefully, understands I'm here in preparation for my upcoming seed implantation, and expertly draws the necessary vials without me feeling the tiniest of pinpricks. (Do I have to tell you I don't look?)

Next is the EKG. I head down to Area J. Area J? Sounds like I'm in Roswell. I give my paper to the receptionist and take a seat. This is a large waiting area. In front of me is the reception desk, behind that a row of treatment rooms. This is not a good place. The people in here do not look healthy, and one in particular is having a serious discussion with a doctor who doesn't seem to be imparting good news. I have to go to the bathroom. I ask the receptionist.

"Across the hall." She smiles.

I recognize her as the woman who accompanies her father to Radiation each morning

"How are you?" I ask.

"Good."

"Your father?"

"Getting along. Thank you for asking."

"The people here are terrific."

She smiles. "Yes, they are."

There are two kinds of bathrooms: one-person jobs (closed and you're dead) and the Megaplex (always room at the inn). This is a Megaplex! I have to remember this lav.

The moment I return to reception and retake my seat, my name is called and I'm directed to a tiny, dimly lit room where I'm to be given an EKG. The tech is Puerto Rican, and as she prepares me for the test she talks to me of her homeland. I learn all about the tiny village where in she grew up and where she returns to each Christmas with her American-born children. From now on, whenever I have suction cups applied to my body, I'm going to think of Gloria Escobar.

I'm back out in reception and need to go to the bathroom again, but first I ask how I can get to B.

"It's right next door to The Breast Cancer Center."

"Breast Cancer Center—where's that?"

"Go all the way down the hall to the main corridor, then make a right."

After my pit stop, I follow the receptionist's directions, and when I get to the main corridor I'm staring at the letter A right above the door marked Breast Center. I pass this door every day on my way to Radiation Oncology and had never once noticed it. The reception area is a good imitation of Grand Central at rush hour. My Radiation Posse is never this large—otherwise, we'd be pissing all over each other. I try to avoid eye contact, but these patients are lovely creatures, and it's hard to look away. To my immediate right is a door marked *Radiology*. After I enter, I see Radiology has its own door. If I were on my game and had simply paid attention, I would have spotted the letter B above the entrance just a few paces to the right of the Breast Cancer entrance.

I sign in. The reception desk services both A and B waiting rooms, and while I wait, I watch women in A sign in and out. Phones are ringing, appointments made, questions answered, calls transferred and connected. I need to ask where the bathroom is located.

"Through that door and to the left."

It's a rat's maze, but I finally locate the one-person job. Closed. I try the knob. Thank God it's empty. I tear at my zipper—pull down my briefs —free my bucking pal, stream splashing the floor on its way to giving the porcelain god a good spritz.

The bursting blue balloon gives no warning and waits for no man.

I'm back in the waiting room and it's more phones ringing and answered, women entering, women leaving, receptionists sneaking snacks, talking small talk. I think of the women in my life—see their faces replace the ones on the other side of the glass.

"Mr. Robespierre."

Now I'm in the X-ray room. I'm instructed to remove my shirt, stand with my back to the machine, and not to move an inch. The person administering the test is a doctor and very professional, his accent distinctly Middle Eastern, and I correctly guess Israeli. A totally non-threatening situation, and fifteen minutes later I'm finished for the day.

I head for the exit and know that never again will I pass Area A without a salute to the staff, to the patients, to their never-ending and most courageous battle.

ROUND 24

GQ Lou and I enter the Chelsea Diner, shake off our wet umbrellas at the door, stomp our soaking feet on the damp carpeting, and head up the aisle. An attractive hostess quickly comes forward and points to a nearby booth. We tell her we like to sit near the coat rack.

I turn to Lou. "And closer to the bathroom."

He laughs, and when Lou laughs it's more contagious than the most virulent virus.

The hostess shows us the booth on the left, two up from the coat rack, the one we normally occupy. We're two happy campers, made even giddier by the sight of our hostess shaking her thang back to the front desk. The Greek manager and the waiters (some Greek, some Hispanic) share our conspiratorial winks and primordial grunts—however, they can't imagine how this involuntary act of lechery makes us feel like normal, healthy guys again.

Lou hangs up his snazzy designer raincoat and wooden-handled umbrella on the coat rack, while I drop my five-dollar number under the table, put my non-designer rain jacket on the seat next to me, and remove my *New Yorker* Magazine and banana from the pockets and put them on the table. I should have followed his umbrella lead, because I've just flooded out the floor under me. I'm in jeans and a sweater while Lou's naturally natty in a dapper, blue wool suit, custom fitted, white shirt, and very plush, powder-blue, silk tie. Lou sits, and before he can settle in, I get up. I have to go to the bathroom. Lou's got to go, too.

"Man, this is getting pretty sick," I grumble as I rise up.

You would think one, maybe two trips to the WC would take care of four cups of water, but noooo—it's got to drag out for two or three hours. Lou's rushing up ahead, nodding in silent agreement. I know this is a complaint that's worn out its welcome (if this is all I have to complain about, I should get down on my knees and kiss the ground), but I'm cold and wet and would just like to sit and relax for a minute.

We head for the restroom. We pass a mother and two-year-old in a corner booth and two teenage Hispanic lovelies cooing in at a table along the back wall, adjacent to the bathrooms.

"Let's use 'em both if they're empty," I say.

When we first came here Lou and I decided if Gals' is taken, plan B is one of us takes the urinal, the other the toilet; if Hombres' is *occupado*, plan C is boys cross swords under the Tampex dispenser. Good news today–both are unoccupied.

"I'll take the ladies," I offer. "I'm feeling frilly."

Lou smiles, nods, probably had the same idea.

As I relieve myself, I'm thinking, *Two guys hurrying for the bathroom together like their life depends on it—no wonder the teens break off their love gazing to give us the eye.* Who else but girlie boys going for a quickie, or druggies making a buy look so desperate? Of course, this is absurd. Nobody's paying us any real attention. In places like this, patrons don't even look up when they're served; they're too busy reading the sports pages or gossip columns. Only me, Mr. Nosey Parker, stares and makes up stories when people pass my table.

I get back a couple of minutes before Lou. While he's away, I order us two cups of coffee, so by the time he's back and looking at the menu the waiter surprises him with his cup.

"Should I drink it?" Lou asks. "The doc says it ain't good for the prostate."

"Sure—coffee's on the list of things that irritate the prostate along with half the stuff we eat, but as long as you have it in moderation, I don't see a problem," I reason.

He orders the lox-and-onions omelet, and I'm in for two eggs up, and about to ask for a side of lox and tomatoes on the side (like the previous times), but Lou beats me to it.

Lou's hesitant to drink the coffee.

"Just drink it, and if you're having trouble, cut down or cut it out. Listen— what's the use of denying ourselves what little pleasures are left to us? Speaking of pleasure," I get up, ". . . got to go again."

On my way back to the bathroom two Hispanic girls eye me suspiciously. I smile and head into the bathroom.

"*Mira, mira*, wanna buy sun Ecstasy?"

I have Pacino down pat as I unzip. "Wanna say hello to my lit-tal friend?" I almost miss the urinal I'm having so much fun doing Tony Montana, and so's my "little friend."

Back at the table I'm listening to Lou complain that he gets up every hour on the hour at night.

"Ng gave me some Aleve," I say.

"Me, too."

"The stuff's great."

"I haven't taken it."

"Why?"

"I don't know."

"What about Flomax? That's helps, too."

"No Flomax."

"You should ask for it, Lou—and get the generic—it's a hell of a lot cheaper."

"My insurance always gives me generic."

"Really? I'm thinking why didn't Medicare or my supplementary AARP do that?"

I love Lou's heavy Brooklyn accent, and if you close your eyes you will absolutely swear he was Tony Soprano's voice coach, only everything Lou intones has a humorous lyricism. This homegrown Bensonhurst vocalization, together with a teddy-bear persona reinforce his likeability, and I want to reach out and remove his pain—not that I'm qualified, considering my own neurosis.

I've got to go again. Lou nods, gets up to join me. We both rush to the back; this time the girls are busy kissing. A group of German tourists argue over the seating arrangement. *Just stay out of the bathrooms.*

Great, empty! I use the little girls' while he uses the boys'.

I'm out first and get a dirty look from a female tourist. Damn it, I wish I knew the German for *transgender*. By the time I get back to my seat it's too late to say, "Ich bin ein Berliner." You can tell I'm feeling better. The booth across the aisle is empty, and sitting on the table is a newly minted copy of the *Daily News,* so I naturally do what all New Yorkers in a diner do—lean across, scoop it up, and stick it under my jacket for the bus ride back across town. The food comes, and so does Killer Kowalski, who sits down in the deserted booth. Before he realizes somebody grabbed his paper and starts to strangle the nearest suspect (me), I pass it over.

"Sorry, I didn't think anyone was here. I just wanted to see the headlines."

"Not a problem."

Killer Kowalski is a wrestler from the Fifties whose chokehold gave me nightmares and the name I attach to any person I believe has equal instincts. This guy isn't a wrestler—just a construction worker or a hired killer. I'm glad he's not pissed.

I slide back to the safety of my booth, stare at the side of lox, and consider stabbing a slab. I also consider eating, but that's rude; then again, Lou does have the habit of taking a long time taking care of business, so I dig in before the eggs get cold. I'm a couple of bites in when Lou sits down.

"They've got to think we're a bunch of cokeheads," he says, as he slides his large frame onto his seat. He laughs. I laugh. I was thinking the same thing.

We both eat, but I notice he seems to be laying off the coffee and the bread, while I'm lathering up my rye toast with the grape jam and almost finish off my first cup of joe. I'm unable to open the butter packet, try hiding my ineptitude, but when I use my teeth all is lost; fortunately, Lou's too much of a gentleman to acknowledge my incompetence.

Lou's a bigwig in high-rise construction, and one of his managerial duties is to ride those open-air elevators up to the top floor and oversee his workers. Obviously, this skeletal area does not accommodate porta-potties, and lack of easy access to the facilities is beginning to cause him concern, but he tells me he'll handle it—and he doesn't have to tell me twice to convince me that when he sets his mind to something, it gets done.

He looks away and stabs a piece of lox. I stare at Lou. He's on to talking baseball and laughing about a play he saw last Sunday. I admire the guy—still looking *GQ*, still making with the jokes.

ROUND 25

I don't have to be at the treatment center until 11:00 a.m., but I'm up anyway. *Try to get back to sleep.* I can't. I'm still ticked off about the change of schedule. Why the hell can't I get my flexibility act together? Was I always so rigid? Is it old fucking age, or is it the cancer? That would be convenient—blame everything on a disease and skate—get a free ride on taking responsibility. I don't think that will wash.

Okay, no big deal. *You're up, so make use of your time. Make coffee—eat breakfast—exercise?* Who said that? *Exercise or get yourself a Santa suit.* There's no one in the room, so how come I'm hearing voices? *Look in the mirror.* I will not. What I need is to cut down on calories. *Calories in, calories out*, that was Helen's mantra and mine when I was co-writing *The Yummy Hunter's Guide* with her. Of course, my road to ruin began with that book.

Let me rationalize and take no responsibility for my actions. We have to test nearly a thousand products over the three years it takes to write and research both editions. Naturally, "test" to any sensible person with a moderate degree of intelligence means *taste*, not *eat*, and that's what Helen and I set out to do, but after a typical day of tasting, Helen would kindly say: "Eric, why don't you take the leftovers home?" This notion appeals to cheapie Eric; only some of the foods I take home—cookies, cakes, candies, chips—is stuff I normally never eat. You can see why one could blame Helen. Okay—it's my own damn fault for taking the stuff home in the first place and worse still, for following the rules of the food hog for which portion control does not exist. Ten pounds later (almost all ugly belly and waist fat), I'm being treated for bad walnuts, and adding injurious behavior to insulting fat, I find myself eating myself silly because I need emotional comfort—and for me that's spelled F-O-O-D!

To make things even worse, one of the side effects of the Lupron is—*you guessed it, Masked Man*—uncontrollable eating urges, and so, all and all, I'm up another sixteen pounds. For those without an abacus, that's a total of twenty-six miserable belly-fat pounds in five fucking years! Talk about your conspiracy theories—my weight gain deserves a senate hearing, or at the very least, a video posting on YouTube.

I suddenly have an epiphany! Everyone knows God divides (beautiful women = dumb stick figures; brainiacs = nerds with pen holders; writers = fantasy dwellers), so why shouldn't he make drugs do the same? Lupron is the perfect example of his handiwork—it turns off your sex glands, but turns on your salivaries, transforming you into the eunuch who eats his refrigerator (this hypothesis does not invalidate my Lupron-as-an-alien-space-craft-theory, for as we all know, we live in separate dimensions).

So, point being—exercise is needed. Walking is out—too damp and rainy. What a wuss I'm turning out to be. Lousy weather never stopped me before. Of course, walking is good for the heart, but let's face it, guys, I could do the two-step from here to Tucson and still wouldn't lose this gut. Push-ups—that'll firm up the belly. Oh, great—so it'll be more pronounced and stick out even further. *Stand up straight, shoulders back, tuck in the stomach.* There's that voice again! Okay—that looks better, only my core is weak and my muscles too tight to do it rigorously unless I want *rigor* to set in. Yoga—back to yoga until I'm flexible, then sit-ups, a regime I follow religiously until this damn prostate business sucks the will to look good right out of me.

Then I ask myself, *Do you want to be the six-pack heartthrob of the cemetery, or have that delicious two-pound bowl of pasta, three big pieces of yummy Italian bread soaked in spicy marinara sauce, washed down with two glasses of Chianti, followed by a tiramisu that brings tears to your eyes?* Hey—da Vinci knew the answer, otherwise "The Last Supper" would be "The Last Workout," and you'd have had twelve apostles breaking a sweat instead of breaking bread.

Yoga—well I certainly have the Buddha in my belly, or the belly of a Buddha, don't I? I have the urge to do yoga today, because I won't be able to do any exercises for at least a week thanks to tonight's second hormone shot. The thought of a second alien spacecraft invading the meditative tranquility of my inner Buddha takes the zing out of my Zen, so I must repeat my postures if I'm to do them properly. This extra effort is either a smart or a very stupid idea, because if I aggravate my herniated disc, lying still on the radiation table will be a bitch.

Fuck it! I have breakfast, two cups of coffee, and make sure I pee even though I don't think I have to—then I'm off by bus to St Vinny's. Despite the pouring rain, the cross-town ride is free of traffic and without any psychosomatically induced urgency problems. *There will be no St Vitus dance on 14th Street today, boyo!* Is this also a sign from above that tonight's Lupron redux will be a harmless walk in the park?

Naturally, thinking of hormones leads me to reflect on my lost libido, and at that precise moment I hear a woman with a pronounced Southern drawl murmur, "This ain't no old-age home on wheels."

Was I thinking out loud, or is that a voodoo woman sitting behind me? As I swing my head up and then around to find out, I spot the object of derision, a group of elderly people slowly getting on the bus. Halfway into my turn (there is no turning back unless I risk herniating another disc) I smile as the woman behind me comes into view, her rising body large beyond any measure of my wingspan. Now fully erect, she somehow navigates a turn and makes for the rear door and even more miraculously squeezes her way out the exit, her Bluetooth flickering brightly in her elephantine ear. I turn back and smile nervously at the old folks who are self-medicating with nonstop laughter. I bet these old geezers are still getting it.

Eric—you poor, miserable son of a bitch—you're jealous. Am not! *Am!* Am not! *Envy migraine! Envy migraine!*

Once I get to the hospital, I enter the outer waiting room, expecting the place to be jammed, but only two patients, both Chinese and both strangers to me, sit quietly in the second row reading their Chinese newspapers. I wave at Barbara and Elizabeth. They wave back. All is right with the world.

Before I can ask my obligatory question, Barbara is on the phone with Radiation—nodding and smiling at me.

"Thanks, Barbara!" I say as I head for the water dispenser.

"Let me tell you tomorrow's time—nine-twenty."

"I'm all over the place this week, aren't I?"

The phones are ringing, and Barbara's got more important things to do than to respond to my whining, no matter how subtle. Elizabeth is doing some whining of her own. Apparently, she sent away for a three-disc collection of 60s classic rock, but one of the discs they mailed is entitled "Caribbean Love Songs."

I mosey over to her desk. She looks up and complains how she's had to wait over two months for the music, but what's even more frustrating is she purchased the music from a local radio station, and when she called they put her on hold, then automatically disconnected her.

I walk around her desk, peer over her shoulder, but quickly turn away should she think I'm looking at hospital records. I suggest she call her credit-card company and cancel payment. She doesn't seem to hear me, or perhaps she's not interesting in replying. Oops—all this chatting and fraternizing is interfering with my frenzied gulping, and if I don't stop my gabbing, I won't finish in time. I edge away, but not before I utter a few words of understanding to show I appreciate her predicament and sympathize with her plight. I knock back the remainder of my first cup, refill a second, and then ask what kind of music she likes.

"All kinds except opera."

"I'm going to make you a few discs."

"You're so sweet, Eric—thank you."

I'm halfway into my fourth cup when Barbara gets the call for me to go in. Instead of gulping down the rest, or trying to finish it off in one long swallow, I take my time between swigs until I'm finished. It's amazing how relaxed and at ease I am. *Well, you've been here five weeks—it's about time you got with the program.* The Voice of Reason has made a point.

I look around and smile, almost out of embarrassment, because the waiting area is now packed with very sad, sick-looking patients, and I'm acting like I'm out for a walk in the park. Shame overheats my body; sweat glands wet themselves. I dump my cup, go into the changing room—no white terry gowns, so I grab one of the flimsy green cotton ones, and wipe myself down as I get undressed in front of my locker. I'm feeling really sad, and tears begin to fall. I quickly dress. I hate to think what would happen if one of those shy, diminutive Chinese women sees me in my BVDs. Speak of the devil, here comes one now. Luckily, I'm presentable. She and I exchange nods.

The treatment waiting room is completely empty. I automatically stare at the watercolor prints that horizontally line the opposite wall. The images at first bring comfort, enter my subconscious, rewire my brain and program me to always pick this seat. *Bullshit*, says my Doomer and Gloomer. Don't the pictures on the wall to my left appeal to me more and resonate with my true sense of beauty? Isn't it also true I obsess about stealing them each day after a treatment, taking one from the wall, putting it under my gown, taking it to the changing cubicle, removing it from its frame, hiding it under my jacket and finally leaving the hospital with it safely hidden from view? I wait for a rebuttal from The Smiley Boys and here it comes: *It's against my nature to steal, but to even contemplate stealing from a place of healing is the height of obscenity, not to mention the consequences of getting caught—punished in ways too horrible to contemplate, but all having to do with death rays and searing melting flesh (thank you again, Steven Spielberg).*

Suddenly a therapist appears, calls out my name, and beckons me into the treatment area. My neurotic distraction is so all-consuming I lose all track of time and place. How wonderful!

I know the drill so, before she even asks, I give her my date of birth, then hand her the CD.

"I'm returning it."

"Do you want to play it?"

"It doesn't belong to me. I borrowed yesterday so I could copy it to my computer."

"Okay."

I follow her into the treatment room. She returns the CD to the stack next to the CD player.

"What would you like to hear today?"

"You choose."

A young woman enters—hesitant and unsure—and right away I figure her for a student. I get up on the treatment table, and under the supervision of the first therapist, Student Girl begins to mechanically raise the table. Then comes the task of getting me into the right position. I instinctively lower my BVDs so my three tattoos are visible. Student Girl points the omnipresent hand-held controller, presses some buttons, and sends signals to the computers in the other room notifying them ROBESPIERRE IS ON THE TABLE. Good! I'm no practice dummy. I'm fucking flesh and blood, and I got me a death ray pointed at me privates. Right? Right!

Student Girl nudges me into position, while on the opposite side, the more experienced therapist expertly tugs on the sheet, showing the newbie the little trick that positions me without having to lift my body. Their coordinated efforts are taking way too long, and I realize the newbie is really a newbie, as in first day—FIRST FUCKING DAY! I try not to panic; evaluate—remember—computers—experienced therapist—not to worry. Right? Right!

"Don't move—we'll do all the work."

"That's what all the women in my life say."

The therapist, then Student Girl make with ha, ha, hahs. *Make' em laugh, always make' em laugh.* I want to reassure the therapist that I know the drill, won't move, show fear, impatience, God forbid annoyance. *Make' em laugh, always make' em laugh.*

There's a few more minutes of pushing and pulling, and finally they get it right.

"Are you taking pictures?"

"We always take pictures."

"I mean the three-sixty set. I was supposed to have them Tuesday, but they forgot—I mean, that didn't happen."

Eric, will you be quiet! Blaming the therapists—are you crazy? Do you want the death ray shot up your ass? Shut the fuck up—don't question—get with the program. These people are professionals. They know what they're doing. They don't make mistakes.

"And the check is in the mail," says Doomer and Gloomer.

I didn't notice Doomer and Gloomer, making their first corporeal appearance, to the left of the treatment table, sitting straight up in director's chairs, pretending to read their Chinese newspaper.

"Not today," the therapist answers.

"Okay." I close my eyes. No pictures—who cares? Right? Right! Just two more days and I'm outta of here. Right? Right!

"Mr. Robespierre—it'll just be a few minutes. Lie still." The therapist turns down the lights and then—*whoosh*—the tomb is sealed.

One one thousand, two one thousand—the treatment hasn't started—what the hell is taking so long? Hold it—they can't start the treatment until the computer makes the obligatory last positioning adjustments. Right? Right! But suppose they forget and start zapping away? And, AND suppose the newbie made a mistake and I'm positioned incorrectly—say two or three inches, enough to fry my blue balloon and turn my piss to steam?

If I could just get up and take that organ of glandular angst and flush the fucker down the toilet.

ROUND 26

SURPRISE, surprise, I'm feeling pretty calm when I walk into Dr. Berman's office. I'm supposed to be the doc's last patient, but I see three or four guys already waiting—then again, this is a group practice, so maybe they're there for another doctor and my wait won't be long. Either way, no biggie; I'm not going anywhere. I check in, find a seat. Nobody looks up. Fear does that to you, makes you hide in a deep, dark, unreachable place, turning even the most friendly of us Humanoids into Voids with *bupkis*, nothing, *nada, rien*, to live for. I'm throwing out smiles, fake ones because I'm also hurting, but my pain has nothing to do with my cancer. All I can think about is Lovely Blonde Nightingale. I miss her. She was with me the last time. She held my hand when I received my CAT and bone-scan results—providing me the courage to begin treatment and get my first hormone shot then and there. If I'm to be totally honest, I've been singing I-Miss-My-Miss-Lovely-Blonde-Nightingale Blues for a few days now, all brought on by the thought of this visit. It's funny how associations work and how they stir up the strongest of emotions—in this case all positive feelings, feelings of love, safety and security, feelings which I'm not feeling now. I'm all alone.

There's no warm and tender hand to hold mine, another life form to comfort my life form—no one at all. I stare into a corner, and there's Lovely Blonde Nightingale in her hot red pants, thick brown walking shoes, and multicolored top, reading a magazine, completely engrossed—yet even at rest, coiled and ready to leap tall buildings at a single bound for me. I look around, to see if anyone is looking, and when I'm sure no one is, I take out a handkerchief and dab the tears away. I feel eyes on me—a receptionist. She looks away in embarrassment—thinks I'm a first-class wimp and scared to death of a little hormone shot. Well, I'm not! I blow my nose as softly as I can, still loud enough to make others look—though thank God not in my direction. I really fucked up and now I'm all by myself. Well, not exactly. Doomer and Gloomer are back, only this time they've shed their corporeal shells and beamed their voices into my head. They slowly take their place under my cranial bandshell and, assisted by my skull's Carnegie Hall acoustics, sound pretty damn good.

"All by myself
Don't wanna be
All by myself anymore
All by myself
Don't wanna live
All by myself anymore"

"Mr. Roseberry?"

I nod, smile, stand. "Robespierre—Robespierre," I reply, the spirit of correction welling up inside me.

"Rose-Pierre —Rose-Pierre."

Obviously, she's not a member of the congregation, so in the spirit of forgiveness, I nod. I dutifully follow the tech into an examining room. It's home to my biopsy and hormone shot.

"Please get undressed to your shorts." She hands me a purple gown.

"Should I leave you a sample?"

"You should always leave a sample," she says, a bit sharply.

I should never have corrected her pronunciation. She could put something in my urine, screw around with the analysis, make me think I need dialysis.

"Your hair looks very nice today," I say.

"Thank you."

I detect a faint smile. *Okay, Mr. Brown Noser, that should do it.* Now I have two choices: Pee and change, or change and then pee. What to do—what to do? Better to be safe than sorry. Right? Right! Sometimes it pays to hear voices. I enter a restroom, well stocked with ready-to-use plastic vials—hurray! Frequent peeing is my life, so to pee on demand shouldn't be a problemo, but it remains to be seen which pressure will rule. I look at the pyramidal stack and remember how frightened I was the first time I left a sample for Dr. Berman. *You've come a long way, Mr. Floppy.* Vial in hand, I step up to the bowl, and like the player who has to sink a free throw to win the game, I take a deep breath, shake my upper torso, and let fly. YES!

I'm back in the treatment room, undressed and ready to go. I'm relaxed. It didn't hurt the last time, so why should it hurt now? Right? Right! What if I have to wait? I brought a book and the latest copy of the *New Yorker*. I don't have to just sit and stare at the neat arrangement of instruments or equally menacing machines just because they're close enough to touch. Would I hear screams? Do they contain the sounds of the tortured? *The Inquisition, the Inquisition . . .* It didn't hurt last time, so why should it hurt now? Didn't I just say that? Well, so what if I did? That's my mantra for today, and I'm sticking to it.

Oops—I make the mistake of looking up at the life-size drawing of my lower innards, which I know is there for educational purposes, but the gory realism scares the bejesus out of me just the same. First off the guy or—should I say, this anatomically correct rendition of the insides of a guy—is one ugly-looking character. Secondly, those reds are too bloody red (no pun intended) and turn my stomach six ways to Sunday. I have to admit he's an eye-catching bugger, one I can't keep my eyes off of, even though I know that would be the wise move. My hands involuntarily cover the family jewels as eyeballs trace an imaginary line from kidneys to bladder to prostate to privates that seem mysteriously less vivid—perhaps created by a God who didn't want to be out-endowed? Let's not go there.

Suddenly, Dr. Berman's in the room.

"How are you?"

"I'm fine."

"That's good."

He's putting on his white latex gloves. The tech must have already laid out the necessary paraphernalia. When did she do that? That's one big fucking needle, and so is the syringe (*better to hold the Lupron II spacecraft, my dearie—cackle, cackle, cackle). Turn away. Close your eyes. In a moment, Dr. Berman will propel Lupron II into your soft tissue.* The only question is—will it join up with its companion ship and together blast away at my cancer cells, destroying them along with my libido, or has Lupron I shot its load (ha, ha) and now lies dormant, its crew waiting to be rescued by Lupron II—OR—are these suicide missions, and once their payloads are dropped, do they disintegrate, evaporate, vaporize, leaving a fat bloated belly as their goodbye gift?

"Tomorrow's my last day of radiation." I didn't plan to say anything, it just came out. Do I think that will somehow stop him from giving me this second shot?

"That's good. Any side effects?"

"Nope. Just some frequency issues."

"Pull down your pants a bit."

"Oh, sure."

"Are you taking Flomax and Aleve?"

"I take one Flomax every evening. I was telling Dr. Ng how expensive that stuff is—he wrote me a script for the generic that costs a lot less."

"I thought it would be another year before one came out."

"Oh—and this tire around my waist, I guess it's from the Lupron."

"You're not getting Lupron—I'm giving you Zoladex."

"Oh!"

What the fuck is Zoladex!? I feel myself about to go into Shit Lockdown.

"Don't worry, the tire should go away."

"Huh?" Zoladex . . . How do you spell . . . ?

"Okay—here we go."

Z-O-L . . .

"You'll feel a little pinch."

"Yep . . . That was nothing."

Look away, close your eyes—yeah, close your eyes. Think of Lovely Blonde Nightingale's wonderful body. There it goes. I feel the pressure. *Keep thinking of Lovely Blonde Nightingale—something specific—her perfectly proportioned ass.* I can hear them—they're communicating with each other:

"How's life back home on Zoladex?"

"Great. Everyone misses you."

"What's it like inside Eric's world?"

"He thinks we're from Lupron."

"Same shit, different day."

"Well, they do spend the big ad bucks."

"Screw Lupron! We're Zoladex, and we make a difference. By the time we're finished, he'll have a tube around him the circumference of our sixth moon."

Foreign-body migraine! Foreign-body migraine!

I feel the needle coming out, Dr. Berman applying gauze, covering it with tape, pressing down on the entry site.

"I want you to apply pressure for about five minutes and then come into my office."

He takes his hand away and leaves. I press down hard and begin counting: *one one hundred, two one hundred, three one hundred . . .* Why do the Zoladexers like pounds of pasta, thick-crusted bread, and high-fat cheese? I've lost count. *Look at your watch.* No good—I don't know when I started. One

one hundred, two one hundred, three one hundred . . . Okay—that should do it. I gingerly get off the table and look down at the bandage. It's a big sucker. Fat belly, fat belly! *Will you stop bitching and moaning?* But this is the flesh of my flesh. *You were overeating before bad walnuts.* Oh—now you're blaming me? *Would you rather be dying of cancer?* What about eating for comfort? *Cry me a river, why don't ya?*

Foreign-body migraine! Foreign-body migraine!

I enter Dr. Berman's office. He's writing. I sit. Wait. Take in the framed diplomas and awards, lock on the two *New York* Magazine Best Doctors of New York covers. I remember when I first looked him up on the Internet and read a slew of patients' remarks, most praising his professionalism and expert care, with only one negative reviewer referring to a cold bedside manner. Cold bedside manner, my ass; this is a doctor who cares enough to pick up the phone and call you with your tests results. You call that cold? Okay, so he's not a joke-telling backslapper. What healer is? I should find that site and add my own two cents, call the malcontent out and whip his sorry ass.

I glance back at my hero. He's fishing around in a side drawer, comes up with a fistful of little white plastic containers.

"Here's some more Flomax."

Drug-company samples: four, no five little containers. What a generous guy. I don't think I'll post this info on the Internet.

"Terrific. Thanks. So—I guess the next time I see you will be on the sixteenth?"

"That's right. You'll see Dr. Ng and me. We work together. We've been doing this procedure for over ten years."

"That's great."

What is it with doctor's offices that bring out these lame remarks? This is why you need someone with you, someone who won't be in doc shock and will be able to respond smartly and ask intelligent questions.

"So, you do the needle insertion and Dr. Ng handles the radiation?" Now this is intelligent.

"That's right."

"Like the biopsy?"

"We don't go in the rectum. I make the three needle insertions under your scrotum, just above the anus. It's much more sanitary that way."

Three needle insertions. This creates some nasty images and freezes up my mind.

"Have you received your pre- and post-op instructions?" he continues.

"Yes."

Do I confess I've read them, but two minutes later totally forgotten everything because they scared the bejesus out of me, or do I just say nothing? I say nothing.

"I want you to disregard what it says about Flomax, and take two the night before and two nightly until I see you after the implants."

"Okay. Uh—what about sex? I'm still by myself, but should I . . . ?"

I know, I shouldn't be coy with someone who's massaged my prostate, but I'm still not going to say *masturbate* out loud. Dr. Berman swivels his chair around, propels himself forward until he's facing a long credenza, opens one of the drawers, and fishes out more samples.

"I don't have any Viagra, but I've got some Cialis. It's a newer version. It doesn't last as long."

"I don't care. I'll take it. This stuff costs a fortune."

He pushes over five sample boxes. Lucky I brought a little plastic supermarket bag with me. It's originally for my umbrella, my book and my *New Yorker*, but it'll be a perfect alternative to stuffing these samples into my pockets. I reach across the desk and shake Dr. Berman's hand. How lucky am I? Here's a doctor, a cancer doctor who is everything a doctor should be: expert in his field, accessible day or night, and above all, painless in the prostate. I really should go on that doctor site and kick that guy's ass.

I'm back on the street. No rain. I could probably walk home, but I won't chance it, not with the Zoladexers orbiting my belly fat. Don't want to do anything to send them off onto a more harmful trajectory, make the belly soreness and discoloration worse than last time, when it turned an area the size of a ham-hock, grey and ash-like, and leached of all its nutrients.

Look—a bus and best of all, there's Circuit City, and you don't even have to pee.

ROUND 27

I'VE forgotten what to do about the hormone bandage, so I decide to put a washcloth over it and take my tub bath cautiously. My legs ache, probably from yoga or yesterday's hour walk, otherwise I'd be taking a shower. I zero in on the insertion site, now swollen and black and blue with growing shades of dark purples and reds; the Zoladexers are on the move, spreading out slowly along my belly's edge, defined by the two pounds of spaghetti for lunch and tuna melt on a football-sized hard roll from last night's pig-out. I wonder if this new band of marauders is in communication with those that flew in on the first invasion, because the terrain has gotten mountainous in the last four months and we wouldn't want these little fellows getting lost and attacking the wrong part of my anatomy. Nobody but me seems to be agonizing over my weight gain of ten or fifteen pounds, depending on my short-term memory, which seems to be shrinking as my belly enlarges. What did Dr. Berman say last evening— fluid retention? Right? Right! Well—maybe I'll just run my finger around it for exercise, safer than jogging around the Central Park reservoir until the paramedics come, don't you think? Oh yeah, he also says something about cutting out junk food, and I reply something about portion size. When he doesn't respond, I mumble something about uncontrollable urges; then it's Lidocaine time, followed by the alien insertion.

I'm worried about my incision (okay, maybe it's not quite an incision) getting wet, so I only fill the tub water up a quarter of the way, just enough to soak my legs, but not high enough to reach the bandage, although I do feel the washcloth covering it getting wet, and that's the signal for me to raise myself up (better to be safe than sorry), a task getting harder and harder with each pound I gain. I take a shower—no boring details necessary, except to say it's another half-assed job and the lower portion of the bandage gets wet enough for me to change it. (Actually, it's only a Band-Aid and a piece of cotton.) I really should clean the wound (okay, OKAY—pinprick), but I'm not dealing with the peroxide pain (sting—it's a sting!); besides, it's not like I can see the damn thing by bending over or positioning myself in front of the bathroom mirror (both of which didn't work the last time), and I didn't buy a hand-held mirror like I promised so it's going to be guess work (again, like last time).

I get a Band-Aid, pull off a tiny piece of cotton from a wad that could clog up the Panama Canal, and paste it onto the small white area surrounded by a sea of black and blue that I figure is ground zero. The cotton is too big for the Band-Aid (I was never good in arts and crafts), so I get another Band-Aid and fasten it vertically. I'm thinking of the scene in *Ronin* where De Niro takes a bullet out of his side, and this image gets me through it. Naturally, I'd rather be Marlowe, but I can't remember him ever getting shot or shivved.

I make two music CDs for Elizabeth, tuck the *Yummy Hunter's Guide* in for Pauline (Replacement Lady has a name), and head out. I get to the front door and it's pouring, so I go back up, put on two layers plus a warmer raincoat, grab a baseball cap and umbrella, and I'm off. So much for not turning on the news or looking out the window—then again, why ruin the surprise?

"Oh, how handsome you look, and how well dressed you are," says Pauline when I arrive.

I have a truckload of witty replies, and an equal stockpile of fawning compliments of my own, but jealous alien invaders have robbed me of my smooth moves, and all I can do is smile shyly and clumsily pull out my gift and hand Pauline the book.

"*The Yummy Hunter's Guide*—how cute. Is that you on the cover?"

"Yes—and my co-writer, Helen Brand."

Pauline rises from her seat, leans over the desk and gives me a peck on the cheek.

"Thank you."

"Yes it's me, and I'm in love again. Had no lovin' since you know when . . ." The Fat Man is in the house.

Eric, step away from the desk before security has to take your jive ass outta here.

Over in the corner I see a good-looking blonde woman who looks vaguely familiar. We greet each other with hellos and a wave of the hand. I hang my coat up and stick my umbrella in the pocket, not worried it will drip because it's safely enclosed in a plastic wrapper the guys at the front door hand me—a real laugh-riot event, because inserting the umbrella into the plastic sleeve reminds us of a penis going into a condom.

I sit next to the blonde, finally remembering that she has to be one who works at the tile company and that I'm temporarily thrown off because she's wearing a different wig

"Louie's not doing well," she tells me. I immediately realize my mistake. It's Joey, GQ-Lou's lovely wife, not the tile lady with breast cancer. "He couldn't pee since last night," Joey continues.

"It's probably a little blockage," I reassure her. "They'll just put in a catheter."

"I know, but it's happened before, and it's making him nuts. The sad thing is, he was so happy before he went to bed, joking and everything."

"I understand. I'm the same way. When there's no pain I'm great, but when there's the least side effect I'm in trouble."

"He thinks he's made a mistake and says he shouldn't have had the surgery. I think maybe he's right. What do you think?"

"Second-guessing yourself will only make you both nuts. The only thing that counts is *now*—and *now* he's in really great hands."

She doesn't look convinced. "He's had emergency surgery before, and each time it takes him longer to bounce back." Her words fall off into silence.

"I'm not sure he needs that—probably just a catheter."

Joey smiles and leans back and looks as if she is starting to believe me. I *knew* I should have been a doctor. If only I didn't have to take chemistry . . . and if pigs could fly, they would be eagles.

I take a moment to look at Joey. Her worried face can't hide her beauty, and she's just as well dressed as *GQ* Lou. I imagine when they're together they make quite the glamorous couple. I'm going to have to fancy myself up if I ever go out with them socially.

Pauline tells me I can start drinking. I get a cup, but instead of standing by the water dispenser, I return to my seat. Joey wants to tell me a horror story concerning an egomaniacal urologist who mistreated her terribly. I already know the story, but I listen anyway.

"Mr. Robespierre, you can go in now."

"Thanks, Pauline." I jump up.

"Tell Lou if he wants, we can all have breakfast."

"We have another appointment—uptown with a surgeon."

"Not a problem. Just give him my best."

She stands. We hug.

"It'll be fine," I say, and actually feel it in my bones I'm right.

I head into the changing room. Something is different. I can't figure it out. I'm still at a loss when I get to the waiting room and sit calmly in my seat, a silly Buddha smile on my face. Thank God everyone has their heads in their papers, completely hidden behind colorful photos and bold Chinese newsprint.

ROUND 28

Friday, May 23, 2008, 6:30 a.m. *Graduation Day . . .*

CELEBRATION time is here! I'm dancing and singing as soon as my feet hit the floor. I'm even ready to take a full bath, soak the living daylights out of my body. So the injection site gets wet? It'll be good for the little devils—that is, if they're still hanging around surface level and haven't already burrowed their way deeper into my tissue. I'm thinking the water will sooth the inflamed tissue, heal the bruising faster, and make the ugly black-and-blue discoloration that has spread to twice its size overnight disappear.

I'm no longer squeamish about removing the bandage, and I do it right after I dry myself off. Boy—the discoloration is really ugly; looks like De Niro's face after the actor playing Ezzard Charles does a number on him in *Raging Bull*. No cotton this time, just one tiny Band-Aid and I'm done.

I speak to Helen, belt out a few lines of "Celebration." I'm on a hormone high. I tell her about Lou and my plans for a graduation breakfast party, and how I've been mulling over the notion of a thank-you-wonderful-people-for saving-my-life gift of two-dozen roses that could be separated out into the various radiation oncology areas. I want to do it today, but because it's Memorial Weekend I'm thinking I could come back on Tuesday. Helen says a better gift would be Munchkins from Dunkin', and they could eat them all today. I immediately like the idea.

The Leo Sayer tune "More Than I Can Say" pops into my head. I can't remember how it goes, so only the title loops through my brain, livening up my moves as I grab a *Yummy Hunter's Guide* for Jane, and then look unsuccessfully for my sunglasses. Finally, I'm out the door, dressed in a neatly pressed blue sports jacket. I wonder if the Fashion Police will give me a commendation?

When I arrive at Dunkin' Donuts, I forget what Helen told me to order, so instead of calling them Munchkins, ask for the Minis. No problemo.

"How many?" The pretty, Indian young lady picks up a bag and turns to look at the display.

"How much?" I ask her.

"$5.99 for a dozen and $9.90 for two dozen."

"Two dozen."

Celebration time, remember!

I'm at Eighth Avenue by 9:05 a.m., and before I turn west on 15th and lose cell service, I call Gillian and wish her a good holiday up in Westport.

"It's my last day, sweetie pie!"

Soon I hear the beep of call waiting, but that's okay, Gil's got to go anyway, throwing me kisses and promising to get together with me next week. I don't need no stinkin' donuts to get me high when I got my darling daughter.

On the other line, it's Lou. He's can't make today, he's just too tired from yesterday's ordeal.

"Not to worry. Just take it easy. We'll get together next week," I tell him.

When I get to the waiting room, the regulars are in their usual seats and Barbara's back at her desk. I give her the Munchkins and ask her to pass them out to staff and patients. She's thrilled and immediately opens the box.

"Thank you! But no can do about the patients—against the rules to give them anything, because they have dietary restrictions. More for us."

I want to say, "More for you," but there's something about radiation that takes the smartass out of you. She selects a Munchkin, calls back into Radiation to cue me in, shakes her head, smiles, nods, and tells me to start drinking. Boy—things are moving fast today. Instead of standing off to the side or sitting down to drink, I drift over to Barbara. On and on I go, like a broken record, telling her for the hundredth time how wonderful she is, how wonderful everyone else is.

Connie and Elizabeth come out of Connie's office.

"Hi, Eric!"

"Hi, Eric!"

"Hi, Connie! Hi, Elizabeth! I brought those for you." Barbara hands them the box of donuts. "It's my last day! It's my last day!"

A radiation therapist appears. "Mr. Robespierre?"

"I've only finished my first glass," I say

"That's all right—as soon as you're done, come in."

"Have a Munchkin."

Elizabeth produces a stack of napkins. The therapist wraps up two for the road.

"See you inside."

"Yep."

The excitement causes me to lose count, so by the time I'm changed and sitting in the treatment waiting room, I've gulped down at least three, maybe four cups. Two regulars, an Eastern European and a Chinese lady, smile when I enter. The Eastern European is waiting for her friend. Initially, I am surprised she's allowed to leave the general waiting area, then I realize it's smart hospital policy, and I wish I had someone here to comfort me.

The Chinese lady has neck or throat cancer. "How are you feeling?" I ask her.

Her English is poor so she uses her fingers to show where the pain is. The Eastern European lady wants to tell me about her own sad thyroid story. She has a thick accent, but her English is good, so I have no problem following her painful journey. In the last two years she's gone from one-hundred-thirty-two to two-hundred-sixty pounds. All her joints ache, making exercise—even walking—painful, and making any weight reduction impossible. She sticks out her fingers to show me how swollen they are and how she can't even wear jewelry. The Chinese woman shows us her fingers and tries to explain something about how they don't work and how hard she has worked these past fifteen years caring for someone, or at least that's what I think she says. When I try to answer her by paraphrasing her remarks, she just continues talking. The Eastern European Woman refuses to look at her and only addresses me, which I think is rude since the Chinese woman engages both of us in her conversation. The woman's friend trudges out, pale and somber, and obviously in great distress. I don't have time to listen to them because I'm called in. The therapist is the same one I saw for the first time yesterday.

"Today's my last day," I say with a smile.

"I don't think so."

My smile freezes. Oh shit, I need extra treatments because my cancer's now responding. Before I can pick out the music for my funeral, she says, "I'm going to check, but I'm pretty sure you get twenty-six treatments."

Student Girl (I guess they didn't fire her) comes over and asks for my info, then leads me in to see Mr. Linear. Accelerator 1.

The first therapist returns, nods. "I was right—you've only had twenty-five treatments."

I feel my flesh tingle. Synapses begin to fire. Speech returns. "What about the pre-screening, or whatever that was? I thought that was counted as treatment number one."

"Nope, that . . . "

I'm not listening anymore. I climb up on the slab of good cheer. *No big deal*, I tell myself, as I listen to the strains of Dinah Washington and add some lyrics of my own.

"Laugh and the whole world laughs,
Cry and they rad your ass anyway"

ROUND 29

THE Fat Man is again in the house—he is me—I am him—I have the mouth—he is the song.

> *"Yes it's me and I'm here again*
> *Had no radiation since you know when*
> *You know I need you, yes, I do*
> *And I'm savin' all my cancer just for you*
> *Need your radiation and I need it bad*
> *Jus' like a dog when he's goin' mad*
> *Hoo-we, baby, woo-we*
> *Baby, won't you give your rads to me*
> *Eeeny, meeny, miney, mo*
> *Told me ya wanted me around Tuesday mo'*
> *Hoo-wee, baby, hoo-we*
> *Baby, don't you let your dog bite me . . . "*

I've already called my cancer posse to arrange a second celebratory breakfast. Last Friday's Felix fête was fun, but wife Judi was out of state, Lou was out of sorts, and I was out a diploma. Like the great Yogi said, "It's déjà vu all over again" as I greet the gals at reception. Barbara immediately informs me Lou's just left. (Judi's the grey-haired, full of fun and high spirited lady I regularly saw in the radiation waiting room; Felix, her loving husband, fellow prostate cancer survivor, and source of strength and inspiration to both Lou and myself.)

"He can't meet you for breakfast—he's going to see another doctor."

I nod, ask the $64,000 question. Tap, tap on the computer keys and she puts me in the queue, then she rings up Radiation.

"When can Eric Robespierre start drinking? Now? I'll tell him."

My last trip to the fancy-dancy dispenser—*yippee-ki-yay!* To celebrate, I vow not to lose count of my cups. Wow, how easy to count up to four without a misstep, and while achieving this feat, even mange to call Felix from the house phone and tell them about Lou. Who says I can't count and make a phone call at the same time?

Judi told me to be prepared to wait after my final treatment for my exit checkup. Since it's also Tuesday and I expect to see Dr. Ng, I really have some serious waiting in store, so I've gone existential by bringing an equally serious profile of Dostoevsky—a mortality wake-up call when one is healthy, but a cold grip of Gloomer and Doomer when you're waiting for Mr. Linear Accelerator 1. I shove the book into my backpack.

"Mr. Robespierre?"

I immediately jump up. Another unfamiliar therapist approaches.

"We're ready for you."

But, there's been a mix-up. When Barbara makes her call she misunderstands, thinks I should start drinking instead of hearing that they want me now.

"I'm sorry, Eric."

"Barbara—no big deal."

As I follow the new therapist out of the room, I recognize her fragrance, realize she's the extremely fetching Chinese therapist I had seen my first week of treatment, whose alluring scent I complimented and discovered to be *J'Adore,* by Christian Dior. Under ordinary circumstances, there's nothing like the scent of a women to create a chubby, followed by the one-eyed snake commanding you to start the seduction process NOW or it will spit fury (ruining your day and your pants)—but when your testosterone level is so low you have to look down to look up, there is serious trouble in River City.

It's two minutes after my last itchy-twitchy feeling. I'm standing in front of my locker, halfway out of my pants, thinking I'm finally back in control, when it starts again.

"Mr. Robespierre?"

I wiggle out of my pants and close my gown as *J'Adore* enters from the door leading to Radiation.

"I hear a rumor this is your last session—congratulations."

I get the feeling this is the standard graduation spiel, nevertheless, it's working, and I find myself getting into the cap-and-gown spirit (okay, there's no cap), or am I just sublimating desires for this adorable creature who, in my almost nakedness, stands before me with smiling eyes that never leave mine?

"I'll see you later, okay?" she says.

"Sure."

I would like to be alone with my *J'Adore,* but the waiting room isn't empty.

I nod at Eastern European Woman, who immediately begins talking. She's remembers this is my last day and congratulates me. I think she says *mazel tov*, so I say *mazel tov*, but I get a blank stare in return. Ooops.

"So, where are you from—Russia?"

"No, no Russian."

"Ukrainian? Hungarian."

She nods, and then struggles to get up, and despite the pain trudges over and sits next to me. *J'Adore* will have to wait until tonight, because Eastern European Woman begins chatting away: Her husband's Northern Italian, a great eater and an even greater cook. Next comes last year's itinerary. (Hungarian Woman has serious bucks to be traveling twice a year to places like Budapest, Pompeii, and Rome, especially when the dollar is sinking faster than the Andrea Doria.) I praise her courage. She places a tender hand on mine and rises as her friend enters. The two women begin a rapid exchange. My father is Hungarian on his mother's side, and I want to tell Hungarian Lady my lineage when she touches my hand because, at that moment, I see my father's smiling face—but it is not meant to be.

"Mr. Robespierre?"

I'm on my feet. *J'Adore*—no, it's Student Girl.

"Mr. Robespierre?"

I follow her into the hall, and before she has a chance, I say, "Nine, thirty, forty-two." I glimpse my photo. "Boy—I don't look like David Duchovny."

No response. Maybe I should go back to my Brad Pitt line?

I pause to greet Mr. L. A. 1—excuse me—Mr. Linear Acceleration 1, and take in his dominion one last time. Student Girl motions me to get up onto the table. She and *J'Adore* maneuver my sveltness up and down and sideways. *J'Adore* is letting the newbie run the show and she's flubbing it, but the real problem is my pillow. It just isn't comfy, and I tell them so—only the more Student Girl adjusts it, the worse it gets. Paininmyhead . . . movenoseslightly . . . teensywinsey . . . deathraycomin' . . . boilsnuts . . . Southernstyle . . . lefteyebrowitches . . . timetosayadiosamigos . . . JosiesOnVacation . . . CDIcopied . . . whysthepillowfuckedup.

Zap number one!

Headwouldexplodedfromthegetgo.

Zap number two!

BareNakedLadiesWhatAGoodBoy.

Zap number three or is it four?

Eyesfollowthinredlineacrossarmature . . . don'tfuckingmove . . . toughitout.

ZZZZZZZZap! IsittheCCfarewell . . . isthistheendofRico?

"Hoo-wee, baby, hoo-we

Baby, don't you let your dog bite me . . ."

Whoosh . . . . I wait until Student Girl lowers the table and I hop off.

"Okey-dokey. Thank you. Have a nice day."

"Have a nice day."

I'm out, wave goodbye to the therapists (I don't see *J'Adore*—unsentimental so-and-so), and I'm off to the bathroom, then changing area, finally back to the treatment waiting room to see Dr. Ng, get my diploma, and sign whatever exit papers I have to sign.

I'm not in the waiting room more than five minutes when Nurse Maureen enters, pretends to pass me by—stops. Nurse Maureen is the head nurse and always has a friendly smile for me from the moment she supervised my admission process to now, here in the hallway.

"Mr. Robespierre, I heard a rumor this was your last day."

I pretend I haven't heard the line before. "Yep. And I want to thank you all for everything." I surprise the head nurse with a cautious hug.

We end our embrace, and she hands me a blue folder. Inside is my diploma.

ST. VINCENT'S

COMPREHENSIVE CANCER CENTER

Department of Radiation Oncology

Congratulations,

Eric Robespierre

This Patient has completed the course of Radiation Therapy with a

high order of proficiency in the Arts of dedication, high courage, tolerance

and

determination in all orders given. We recognize this as an Honorable

Achievement,

and would like to congratulate you on a job well done.

Radiation Oncology

Patient Care Staff

2008

How cool is this? When Judi told me about her decision to decline her diploma, saying she doesn't want reminders of the treatment, I thought, *Good idea*—besides, how cheesy is this ritual? But then something comes over me these last days (call me sentimental), and I want the diploma. So kill me (wrong choice of words), but I'm proud I completed my course of treatment. I know I'm doing the right thing, because I see now how this rite of passage is important to the staff so I'm just as excited as Maureen when she plays her little game and hands me my sheepskin. I give her another hug, this one a little more adventurous. *My, what a nice, voluptuous body you have, Nurse Maureen. Better with which to squeeze my patients with, Mr. Robespierre.* We break apart, and I shake her hand. She's smiling. I wonder if she can read minds.

"Oh, by the way, do I see Dr. Ng today?"

"No. See Connie, she'll set you up for your next appointment."

I easily find the right exit door (it took me five weeks), and I'm in the waiting room. I say goodbye to Elizabeth and to Barbara. Elizabeth stands and gives me a hug. Barbara tells me Lou couldn't wait. I nod; no need to remind her she already gave me the message. I'm disappointed—I want to celebrate my graduation. I scan the room for someone recognizable, but they're all strangers. Connie comes over, hands me an appointment card. I give her a quick, impersonal hug. I don't want anyone to think I'd use my condition to get a few cheap feels, although the thought does cross my mind. My friendly gatekeepers are busy with new admissions, but they still have time for me.

"See ya when I see ya!" I say. I know they know the movie because they always laugh and give me the Brad Pitt salute.

Out in the street I take a deep breath. It's a gorgeous day. I'll walk home. For the first time in a long time, I'm absolutely sure I won't pee in my pants.

ROUND 30

I'M getting grief from Helen. She doesn't like the idea of no one going with me to the hospital, nor waiting there until I have to leave.

"It's enough for Steve to come by at 12:00 p.m. to pick me up," I say incredulously.

"No, it's not."

Helen wants to come in, but she's got a full day with clients at her gym. I forbid her to even think about it.

What about Gillian?, she asks.

"Gillian—of course why didn't I think of her!"

My darling daughter has already volunteered. I'm usually too proud to accept her help, or ask for it, using her busy life as an excuse, but now I really need her loving hand. Nick would be there for me in a second, but he's a freelance director with jobs that frequently take him out of town, so unless Gil doesn't think she can handle it, I'll leave him out of this.

I give it another hour before I risk waking my daughter so early on a Saturday morning. She's excited by my request. I tell her she can have my room and I'll sleep on the couch, but she decides she'll stay with my ex and sleep in her old room. Even though the apartment is a few blocks away, I'm a little concerned about her walking over at 5:30 a.m., but after checking Monday's expected sunrise, I'm relieved it'll be nearly light out when she comes over. It's still undecided whether Gillian will stay at the hospital, or leave and then return around twelve. I'm happy with whatever decision she makes. I call Steve, and he's okay with the new arrangements. Maybe it's me, but I detect a note of dejection, so I tell him if I buy the farm, he still gets the pimpmobile. This leads me to thinking about what life would be like without me—not a good place to go, with aliens orbiting my insides and rads heating up my family jewels to levels not seen since Three Mile Island.

ROUND 31

OKAY, let's look at the sheet for the thousandth time.

Pre-Operative Instructions:

Two weeks before surgery, no aspirin, Advil or anticoagulant agents such as Coumadin or Vitamin E.

Check!

So why do I keep re-reading it? *Because, Eric, you want to discover that you didn't follow the directions, have to call St Vinny's and cancel.*

Check!

Bowel Preparation: Two days before surgery drink one full bottle of citrate of magnesium. Eat low-fiber, light food (pasta, fish, chicken, white rice). No fruit or salads, grain bread, veggies, red meat.

Check! Check!

One day before surgery, you are permitted to drink only clear liquids–broth, tea, apple juice, Jell-O. No milk, no coffee.

Check! Check! Check!

I make tea and for lunch broth, but I want a goddamn muffin—a blueberry one from Graceful Foods—and one of their large cups of French Roast.

It's Sunday, for shit's sake, and on Sunday I always treat myself to a muffin and coffee at Graceful Foods. *All right, make the tea, then let's go out and take a walk.* Wait—shouldn't I conserve my strength? What a pussy idea. I'm fine. That citrate of magnesium cleaned me out, and I'm full of pep—vim and vigor, piss and vinegar. Okay—maybe I'm exaggerating a little.

11:00 a.m. It's a nice, warm day, with a chance of thunderstorms late in the afternoon, but I don't care. Weather isn't of interest to me; I'm not going anywhere. No outdoor events: lunches, afternoon aperitifs, long walks along the East River, Battery Park, Central Park. Why? Because—I am The Turtle. That's right, I am no longer human. I am The Turtle, and I can hide in my little carapace—safe and secure, I am. If I am to venture out, it's a cautionary path I choose, completely out of harms way. Look—there's a farmers' market at the 14th Street side of the Oval, but The Turtle isn't going anywhere near it, nor toward the freshly baked breakfast muffins, farm-fresh juice, milk, home-brewed coffees, and herbal teas, their tantalizing aromas wafting across the green.

Just as I get to First Avenue, I spot Steve across the street. Traffic obscures my view, but when I reach the other side he's gone. (What do you expect? I'm The Turtle). I scan the avenue, once, twice—nothing. He has to be in the grocery store. I look through the window—no Steve. I turn, look up and down the avenue again—nothing. He's got to be in the bodega.

The tiny store is a warren of shelves packed and stacked to the ceiling. Suddenly, my pal emerges from behind a wall of Fruit Loops.

"Hey, Steve!"

"Hi, Eric!"

This is good, very good. We'll bitch about politicians, talk baseball, ogle the nubile lovelies on the Oval and, for an hour of so, The Turtle will come out of its shell.

It's 10:00 p.m.—do you know where your rectum is?

Use one Fleet Enema the night before your surgery (approximately 6:00 p.m.).

Take Cipro the night before surgery (approximately 9:00 p.m.),

and drink one full glass of water afterward.

Do not eat or drink after midnight.

Yep—more instructions—ones I forgot to mention, and I know why. The enema! Yuck! I took the Cipro, but I put off the Fleet until now. *10:00 p.m. Do you know—?* I know, I know . . . I'm just no fan of shoving stuff where the sun don't shine.

That's funny. With all those rads, it's probably brighter than Macy's window at Christmas.

Round 32

I'M pretty calm, however, I've got the disturbing feeling that lying beneath the surface of my consciousness is a massive electrical grid, ready to short circuit and send my body into uncontrollable spasms. I'm Gyrating Man, or will be. This is different than Flash Man, able to incinerate at a single rad, or Splat Man and his rupturing blue balloons. I'm glad I'm not feeling like Drowning Man, because I have to take a tub bath and soak my sore bottom. If you're wondering how the Doomers and Gloomers transform me into these heroes of self-destruction, ask the Smiley Boys, who are supposed to keep the zing in my Zen.

I towel off and do a quick shave (don't want to turn into Gyrating Man with a razor in my hand). I dress in jeans, white polo shirt, sneakers, then for the hundredth time (in the last ten minutes) scan my pre-implant instructions, and realize that (yet again), I've done everything as instructed, and have absolutely no excuse not to go through with the procedure.

I stuff the instructions into the appropriate envelope, which already includes the single sheet relating to my personal history that must accompany me to the hospital, when I decide they warrant another look, in the off chance I miss something that will save me.

Allergies—*none*—check. Operations: insert *tonsils and adenoids*—check.

Don't do it! What say you, don't look at the next pages? MEDICATIONS AFTER SEED IMPLANTS. *Cipro, Flomax Steroid Medrol Pack,* and very specific instructions about when, how many, and with what I can take it. Sure, the steroids come with some scary side effects, but nothing like the info that waits for me on the next page. *Don't do it!*

INFORMATION FOR PATIENTS TREATED WITH PERMANENT PROSTATE IMPLANTS

IMMEDIATE POSTOPERATIVE SIDE EFFECTS:

1. Slight bleeding beneath scrotum

2. Blood in the urine

3. Bruising and tenderness between the legs

During the procedure, needles and other instruments are used to place the seeds into the prostate glad. This often causes temporary local tenderness. If you should experience severe pain or severe bleeding, you should call your urologist.

If you cannot pass urine after the procedure, a catheter is placed into the bladder and is removed 1–2 days later. It is normal to have some blood in the urine, which will drain from the catheter. If it becomes severe and/or is associated with large blood clots, call your urologist

There's more, but I have a sudden need to *rendezvous* (yet again) with the porcelain god. What irony. For once a nervous shit will be a good thing, so why am I sitting in the dark, my exposed legs cold and dotted with goose bumps? Maybe I should call Ira again? No. *It will be a walk in the park*—his exact words.... *"Fear is the mind-killer, fear is the mind-killer."* I'm sorry Marlowe's not here, but I sent him over to escort Gillian.

I check my alarm clock, not my watch, because I'm not taking it or my Tibetan prayer bracelet, given to me (by way of a wealthy contributor) by the Dalai Lama. It's 5:45 a.m. I call Gillian. She sounds dead to the world, but tells me she's on her way out. I go around the house turning off lights, cleaning up a stray dish and drink glass. I make sure the bathroom's clean. I can't have my daughter bringing me home to a dirty house. Plus, cleaning calms me down. Maybe I can tidy up around the hospital?

I stare at my hands—not shaking—a good thing. I look out the window. It's light out. Gillian will be safe. Marlowe should have stayed with me. *"Fear is the mind-killer—fear is the mind-killer."*

I'm in front of the house now. I check the time on my cell phone—6:00 a.m. I look toward 20th Street and see my darling daughter approaching. We hug in one long, emotionally uncompromising embrace. Oh, how joyful that feels, so generous that sweet tranquility. I don't see Marlowe, but I know he's near.

We make small talk as we walk through Stuyvesant Town toward 14th Street. I'm figuring if we can't catch a cab, we can always take the bus. Gillian also suggests taking the L train that'll let us off at Seventh Avenue and 14th Street. No problemo—a cab rolls up when we get to 14th Street. Our destination is 170 West 12th Street, but I tell the cabby 12th and Seventh will be fine. We cross 14th in record time, and we're at the hospital by 6:20 a.m., a full hour and ten minutes early. Gillian reaches for her wallet, but I gently put my hand on her wrist. I thank the driver for the "smooth and comfortable ride" (my exact words) and tip him an extra buck. I'm exceedingly nice. That's the way I get when I think I'm about to die or be seriously maimed. There's a shrine on the dashboard, so I figure I'm in a holy place and maybe The Big Guy's listening in. When I get out I see it isn't a shrine, but an ornate air freshener.

I spot a dark blue canopy jutting out and figure that's our destination. We head toward the canopy. 170 West 12th Street. All right then! We spin through the revolving door to be greeted by a sleepy uniformed guard. I suspect he's Indian and wish I could flash my prayer bracelet, establish a rapport, maybe even get a bow and a prayer. (I screwed up in the cab earlier, but I know for sure that this is a Gandhi-*Landsman)*. Before I can open my mouth, he asks my name.

"Eric Robespierre. I'm here for . . . " I glance at the sheet glued to my hand. " . . . The Ambulatory Surgery Department, The Spellman Building—fourth Floor?"

He smiles, turns and points. Why did he ask for my name? I don't see any sheet. Could he have possibly memorized the list?

He's giving us directions: "Head to the end of the corridor, make a left at the chandelier, take the elevator on the right to the fourth floor, make a left, first door on your right."

I nod. I hear it all, repeat it and follow the directions, but I'm counting on Gillian to remember, because I know I'm going to get lost.

At the end of the hall is an imposing marble statue of Cardinal Spellman, the former head of the New York City Archdiocese. This is a good omen, even for a Jew, because back in the early Fifties when I was a little boy, the very same cardinal blessed me, in Columbus Circle, as part of some outdoor ecumenical event my mother and I came upon as we exited Central Park. This is a very good sign.

We get to the fourth floor, but miss the first right after the first left, however, fortune smiles upon us and we meet a nurse who immediately sets us straight. We enter a large waiting room and proceed to the reception desk, where a very handsome but bleary-eyed twenty-something checks my name against his list, points to a door, and tells me to head there. He's all business and not the least bit friendly. The Kindly Ones at the Cancer Center have spoiled me. Too bad they don't perform the surgery there.

Gillian isn't allowed to come with me, but she can wait here, or head out and return when the procedure's done. Twenty-Something hands her a numbered card, tells her he'll call the number when I'm ready to be picked up. Gillian's not sure whether she'll stay in the neighborhood or go back home. I tell her I should be out by twelve, but maybe, to be on the safe side, she could be back by eleven-thirty. This is my way of signaling I don't want her to leave. I think she gets the message because she gives me another hug, this one even more emotional than our morning meet-and-greet.

I bravely head straight for the frosted-covered door into hell—even though the signage reads *Ambulatory Surgery Unit Pre-Op*. They can't fool this homey.

I'm immediately facing a wall of self-contained cubicles separated by curtains that can be drawn for complete privacy, immediately reminding me of the Atlantic City ICU my dad ended up in after he collapsed in his apartment several months before he died, back in that horrible year of 2002. Now it's my turn to get sick and die. I force myself to smile. I'm not my father. I'm not going to die. This is a walk in the park. That's what Ira said, so it must be true. *Remember—"fear is the mind-killer—fear is the mind-killer"*

I suddenly feel cold and clammy—my black cloud of depression is in the building. Before I lose consciousness, the back page of the *Daily News* stares me in the face, then Marlowe appears out of the noxious swirl.

"Hey, pally, if you're gonna throw a joe, don't expect me to pick you up off the floor."

Square, concrete jaw you could break your hand on; high forehead with a couple of blood-red, jagged, crisscrossing scars over half-moon brows; close-cropped, wire-brush grey hair with flecks of white; broken nose set too often, too carelessly; cold blue eyes willing mine to focus. Glad to see my ordeal hasn't changed him.

"It's a walk in the park," he says.

"Yeah," I say, with the hardness of a Frozen Chosin Gyrene. I'm not seeing any steel, so I don't reach for my rod. "So I've heard."

"After it's over, let's dangle—head over to my place and gargle."

I don't say anything. I'm no rube from the cube.

The stall directly facing the entrance is empty, but I'm eyeing the one to the left where Marlowe's sitting, reading his *New York Daily News*. I keep moving and he doesn't look up. I'm cool.

I glance further to my left, spot the nurses' station and a bunch of nurses and techs chitchatting away. I walk over, an eye on the group, the other taking in the cubicles. Most are empty, but one or two are occupied with patients being readied for their procedures. I see an elderly Hispanic woman, a middle-aged Indian lady, both in obvious discomfort, but most disturbing is the fact that all are surrounded, comforted by friends or family. What's with that?

I get to the nurses' station, stand there like The Joker, a forced smile pasted to my face. Finally, a sphinx impersonating a nurse acknowledges my presence. I state my name, hand her the ubiquitous Personal Information Form. She checks it against the scheduled procedures, then instructs a tech to lead me to a cubicle where I am to wait until the arrival of a nurse. I read *Mary S., RN* on her nametag. I give Mary a big 10-4, but she's already taking a phone call and doesn't respond to either my thank-you or my pasted smile.

I'm still feeling no love, and my *Shining* rendition of "Here's Johnny" is just millimeters away from hacking its way to the surface. I get the premonition we're headed for that first vacant cubicle I passed when I entered the floor—*oh, how right you are, Carnac the Magnificent!*

The tech ushers me into my cubicle. "A nurse will be with you shortly. In the meantime, fill this out." She produces a two-page hospital form and a pen. "I'll be back with a gown for you to change into and a garment bag for your clothes."

Marlowe appears. "Come on, pally, don't make me give you the Broderick— dip into the ink and answer the bell."

"Easy for you to say, but did you catch that West Indian chill?"

"Your imagination, pally."

"Cold shoulders, that's all I'm getting, Marlowe. First from Reception Guy, then Station Nurse S., now East Indian Tech Person."

"Suppose you think the frosty window means something?"

"Entrance to hell is what it is."

"That a fact?" Marlowe grins. "Don't let these highbinders do you ugly. Use the Chandler charm, kid. Remember how we turned it on in the bookstore?"

"You call putting on fake specs and asking for a bogus first edition in a nerdy voice charm?"

"Hey kid, did Dorothy Malone give us the eye?"

"Okay—I'll give it a whirl."

West Indian Tech, the form and ballpoint pen still in her outstretched hand, is staring at me.

"Hi, I'm Eric Robespierre. It's a pleasure to meet you. I really love your accent." I relieve her of the form and the pen and give her my biggest Marlowe smile and winky-dink, but noooo—*bupkis*, nothing, *nada, rien*; she just stares at her clipboard, then turns her back on me and walks away. Maybe it's the frigid air that's frozen her West Indian ass shut? Marlowe just shakes his head.

"That's the best you could do, pally?"

"Yeah, well short a shovin' a gat down her throat, like to see you do better. I'm not taking anyone's guff any longer, I can tell you that."

I take a seat on the large and very comfortable recliner. The first page of the hospital form appears to be a duplicate of the one I brought in. The second page is something entirely different and makes me want to bolt. This is the stuff about giving your permission to let the doctors remove your skull and use it for a dashboard display, or the incomprehensible lawyer lingo absolving everyone including the statue of Cardinal Spellman from blame should they take out your left kidney when you're scheduled for a eye exam. Hey—I don't need a Captain Midnight Decoder Ring to read between the lines here.

Calm yourself—it's a walk in the park . . . it's a walk in the park—"fear is the mind-killer . . ."

I'm sorry I didn't bring something to read: a book, a newspaper, my last will and testament—anything to distract me from Doomer and Gloomer and their Army of Angst. *Boots on the ground now—taking the hospital stairs two at a time now—gung-ho to bore through my skull, breach the synapses now—neurotic download—neurotic download!*

A cleaning person, humming softly as she slowly mops the floor in front of a door marked *Bathroom*, distracts me. She glances in my direction and smiles. I return the good cheer. I'm feelin' the love. Normally, the thought of a bathroom so conveniently located comforts me, only now it's doing the opposite. *Okay Eric, just relax. Maybe you're not nervous; maybe it's your body telling you to make one last clean-your-insides-out.*

I rise and head to the b-room. I'm in a collision course with two stern-looking nurses armed with clipboards. I screech to a halt.

"Hi!"

"Hi!"

"Hi!"

I watch them shake, rattle, and roll toward the nurses' station, then, sensing someone approaching, I hurry into the bathroom before I lose out.

The bathroom's clean and spacious, but I'm wise to its dangers so you can bet I'm not sitting down on this breeding seat of infection until I thoroughly cover it with the appropriate toweling; no small trick, because I'm never able to easily separate the middle and place the U-shaped paper properly on the seat. Today, shaky hands make the job twice as difficult.

I'm back in my cubicle, watching a new patient arrive. She appears to be in her late sixties and she moves cautiously, obviously in pain, helped by supporting relatives on either side who treat her with the loving care she deserves.

"All by myself . . . I'm all by myself . . . "

Boy, if I could carry a tune, I'd be belting this one down the hall instead of whispering it into my navel. So—can you tell me why Gillian isn't allowed to be here to keep me company, comfort me until I have to go up to surgery?

The West Indian Tech returns with a full-sized black garment bag. She hangs it up on a cubicle wall. She also brings me a green hospital gown and a pair of grey hospital socks. I'm to put all my belongings in the bag, get into the gown and socks, but first she takes my temperature and blood pressure. Temperature is taken in the ear—yep—you heard me right, in the ear with a sleek beige-colored gismo. After getting a reading (she doesn't look as if anything's wrong), she removes the plastic rubber tip from the gismo's needle attachment and tosses it into the wastepaper basket next to my recliner. She uses the old-fashioned pressure cup to measure my BP. I look away. I'm nervous as a cat on a hot tin roof and I know my pressure's going to be crazy-high. Finished with her tasks and again showing no expression (either I'm alright, or she just doesn't care, or I'm going to die and she's run out of tears for today) the West Indian Tech leaves, but not before making a move to close the curtains. I make a command decision—I decide not to draw the curtains. Sure—the distractions are frightening, but leaving me alone with my morbid imagination is more so. I remove my sneakers, socks, put on the soft, ankle-high hospital socks I remember wearing when I went for my bone scan. This sends me off into a Lovely Blonde Nightingale reverie. I immediately terminate these sacred memories or I will start sobbing and everyone will misinterpret my tears for fears.

Off go the pants, shirt, and briefs. I stick my wallet and house keys into my sneakers, then place the Pre-Implant Instructions in with my pants and zip everything up. Maybe I should have explained why my BP is out of whack—they've got to know how nuts patients get. Right? Right!

I notice there's no lock on my clothing bag, but they must lock it up. Right? Right! A nurse stops in front of my cubicle, smiles.

"Hi, Mr. Robespierre."

Smiling Nurse sits down on the little chair next to my recliner. Her name is Alice. Alice looks to me to be of Irish ancestry. She's in her mid-forties and judging by the absence of a ring on the lassie's left hand, unmarried. Nurse-Alice-With-The-Smiling-Face immediately generates warmth and caring, and I feel my heart rate quickly slowing down. I want to look at my hands. I don't think they're shaking, but just in case, I keep my eyes level with hers.

Guess what Nurse-Alice-With-The-Smiling-Face wants? To ask me the same questions I answered on my Pre-Operational form. Sure, I could bitch and moan, tell her to take a look at the stinkin' forms I've already filled out and just handed her. But you think I don't know she may be in the operating room this morning, turning up the wrong knob, handing over the wrong size scalpel, all because I unloaded on her about these stupid stinkin' forms. I take a breath. I'm happy to help. More than happy—I'm jumping-over-the-moon ecstatic.

Nurse-Alice-With-The-Smiling-Face finishes taking info, then puts a gentle hand on my arm.

"Who will be coming to pick you up?"

"Gillian—my daughter. My daughter's coming."

I want to tell her only a terrible misunderstanding prevents her from being here now—that we love our elders—that we have the same family values as Chinese and Hispanics. Nurse-Alice-With-The-Smiling-Face jots down Gillian's phone number (which I don't have memorized and must look up in my cell phone that I realize I've been clutching in my left hand ever since I arrived.)

"Gillian—oh, that's such a pretty name." She smiles. I smile. Well, this is good—not dancing-in-the-aisles good, but definitely sitting-by-a-warm-cozy-fire good.

Does her hand linger just a mite little longer on my arm than is proper? I must admit I do look hot in this hospital gown. I think the green picks up the green in my skin. Maybe it's my cool? Women like men who have that detached, distant, ice-water-running-through-his-veins look. It's the aura of mystery that draws them to us. Mr. Mysterioso—that's me all right. Why, I hardly react when she puts her hand on my arm. No rude bulge coming up from my groin, foaming mouth, bug eyes, lascivious smile—macho-man speak. I'm cool as a cucumber, and for someone whose cucumber is recumbent, that's a trick.

She's talking to me. "Has the anesthesiologist arrived?"

"No."

"Well—he should be here shortly." (Slight pause.) "Mr. Robespierre, I'll keep a special eye on you, don't you worry." Nurse-Alice-With-The-Smiling-Face winks with such determination I suspect she has "tic douloureux," a nervous affliction I exhibit when I also tell a boldfaced lie, although I don't believe mine is as noticeable.

I feel my phone pressing against the flesh of my palm. I relax—I don't want to break the only link I have with the outside world. I flip through contacts list. Who can I call? Well—it's 6:45 a.m., and that doesn't leave me with many choices, does it? Out of the corner of my eye, an ominous shadow moves in my direction.

"Mr. Robespierre, I'm Dr. Aaron Kopman. I'm your anesthesiologist. Can I sit down?"

"Sure."

"So—have your doctors come in to see you?"

"Nope. Still sleeping, I bet."

We both share a chuckle, or what passes for one under the circumstances. I feel at home with this guy, whose easy-going manner is even more calming, more reassuring than Nurse-Alice-With-The-Smiling-Face's lustful grip. (Okay, maybe it isn't so lustful.)

I sense Kopman is a *landsman*, and I want him to immediately know that, despite my goyisha name, I'm one, too. Why? I have a silly, misplaced notion he will treat a fellow Jew Boy with extra special care.

"I'm feeling a little *shvach* and *farblondzhet*," I say.

That should do it—Yiddish expressions that right away scream in our own secret language, I MAY BE IN A CATHOLIC HOSPITAL, BUT I'M FUCKING JEWISH, SO REMEMBER THE HOLOCAUST. No reaction — so I hit him with:

"I know my name's not Jewish, but I am, and so was my dad and his grandfather, but I'm figuring before that it was changed because there weren't many Jews in France during the French Revolution—you want me to sing my *haftorah*?"

He smiles, nods indulgently, as if encountering a babbling idiot. "Didn't Robespierre cut off people's heads?"

"Yep, but I promise I won't do that to you." I can't stop myself.

He feels my pulse. Nods approvingly. "So, you ready for this?"

"I'd rather be on The Riviera."

"Me, too—let's go."

"Don't tempt me."

More chuckles. "You mind if I take your blood pressure?"

What—I'm going to say no?

"So—what did you eat this morning?"

Is this a trick question? "Nothing—last thing I had was the Cipro and a glass of water—about 9 p.m. last night."

"Good." He also seems satisfied with the readings on the blood pressure gauge. I must be calming down. "No allergies, heart problems, nothing we should be concerned about?"

Does the "we" include me, because if it does—I HAVE CONCERNS!

"Nope, just an innocent heart murmur."

"When did you find out about that?"

"When I was a kid."

"Not anything to worry about."

Well—that's a relief. So I make with the funny. "I'm glad to see someone my age still has a job." What I really want to say is something more serious as in, *You look like you've got the experience and you're expert enough to make sure nothing happens to me.*

He laughs at my funny.

"I lied on my resume. They think I'm only twenty-five."

"I can see that." We both ha-ha some more. I don't know about *him*, but *I'm* suddenly feeling better.

He's got a gleam in his eye as he slowly pushes his large frames up, easy like, reminiscent of the Duke. I'm waiting for "Saddle Up, Pilgrim" but get instead . . .

"I'll be back in a while to take you to the surgery. Just relax, Eric, it'll be fine."

"How long do you think it will take? I told my daughter to pick me up around 12:30 p.m."

He looks at his watch. "You're scheduled to go in at 7:30 a.m. I say you'll be out by 10:30 a.m. to 11:00 a.m., and ready to go home by 12:00 p.m."

"Okay."

As soon as he leaves, I dial Gillian and get her on the first ring. She didn't go back home, she's hanging out in a local coffee shop. I let her know what the anesthesiologist said, adding , "Maybe, just to be safe you'll be here around 11:00 a.m. to 11:30 a.m.?"

"Absolutely, I'll be there. How are you feeling?"

"Great. I feel fine." I see Dr. Berman approaching. "Ooops, here's Dr. Berman—I'll see you later."

"Okay, Pops. I love you."

"I love you, too."

Always the distinguished, bespoke patrician, Berman now appears godlike in his green surgical gown and cap. I gaze at the familiar, yet disturbingly different figure: this guy's really a surgeon—he's really going to cut me open (all right, put holes in me) and shit—something may go the fuck wrong—and I'm gonna die!

He's talking, I'm answering.

"Yes, I took the Cipro. Yes, I took two Flomax."

He pats me on the shoulder. "I'll see you in a little while, then."

I want to say something profound, make him love me more than anyone else in the world—but nothing comes to me.

I hardly have time to catch my breath when Dr. Ng appears and sits down. He's carrying a little metal cylinder I figure to be the lead-line container that holds my radioactive seeds.

"Ahh, the other half of the deadly duo."

He smiles at my Batman reference. He's also in his green surgical garb, but he's looking more himself than Dr. Berman. Why is that? Berman's the surgeon, the cutter, the hole puncher, and Dr. Ng is only the planter, the seed pusher; at least that's how my brain must be registering them, assessing them, filtering them, listing them on a scale of one to ten as to who is most likely to kill me during this procedure.

"How are you feeling?"

"Great."

"Good."

I point to the container. "Are those my seeds?" Suddenly, I'm feeling pride of ownership. How sick is that?

"Yes."

"How many in there?"

"One hundred and thirty-eight, but I may not use them all. It depends on the size of your prostate. I always bring extra just in case."

I want to say something to make him love me most—in case he forgets to add the right amount of seeds and over-radiates me, burns my prostate, bladder and rectum to ashes, or under-radiates me and allows cancer cells to live and be well so they can take a road trip, a couple of day trips, or if they like it stay longer, perhaps even a permanent resettlement in one or more of my vital organs. I want to say something about my prostate as it relates to the size of my penis, but I'm too frozen with fear to be clever, so I do what comes naturally in moments of pending doom—suck up.

"It's good to see you—thanks for everything—you're terrific!"

Dr. Ng smiles, rises, and leaves with his canister of death. Damn—I should have flattered Berman like I just did with Ng. *Shit, shit, and double-shit!* Okay—I still have time in the OR—no—they'll probably shoot me up with something long before I get there. *Shit, shit, and triple-shit!* I'm once more in Shit Lockdown as I watch Dr. Ng walk to Berman, who's standing by the door. They start to chat. I hope Ng's telling Berman what a great guy I am and not comparing hangovers or bitching about Medicare nickel-and diming them to death.

I remember something I read online: "During the procedure, needles and other instruments are used to place the seeds into the prostate glands . . . " I knew I wanted to ask them about "the other instruments"—like what the fuck are they, and why don't you name them? Huh? Huh!

"Will you relax, pally?"

"Oh, it's you . . . "

I will myself into what I can only describe as a state of rapid eye shock (RES), not to be confused with rapid eye movement (REM). I know it sounds paradoxical, but as my blinkers furiously take in the disturbing images, my brain refuses to let them into my optic nerve. Fortunately, my soundless babbling comes to a screeching halt as Dr. Kopman lumbers into frame.

"All right Eric, time to go."

"Huh...?"

"I'm going to walk you over to the OR."

"Huh . . . ?" I get up, walk with him. "Huh . . . ?"

My mantra of the moment—*huh, huh, huh?* We enter the hall. *Why are they making me walk? Don't these people watch movies about death row?* We make a left and pass the waiting-room doorway, where, just a few footsteps away, Gillian may be sitting. For an instant I consider breaking out, finding my darling daughter, embracing her in one giant bear hug until security forcibly returns me to Dr. Kopman. The hallway is empty. For some reason I thought the operating rooms were on another floor.

"So, how long have you been doing this?"

"Thirty years."

"I'm glad this isn't your first." I want to add, *I hope this isn't your last,* but a hospital worker enters the hall and I focus on him, wondering is he a doctor, nurse, tech, or psycho in disguise—like that nut job in *The Hospital* who declares himself the "Paraclete of Kavorka." *Oh great, canisters of oxygen! Keep your eyes straight! See no evil! See no evil!* I focus on the sound of my shuffling feet and *wham*—Sean's in the house and I'm dead man walking. Then a blaze of greenish-blue light beckons me in.

I can't get it out of my head how totally bizarre this is—strolling into the OR, fully conscious and completely aware you're walking into the *pissoire.* How about flying high into the sky with an IV in my arm? *It's a bird—it's a plane—it's Eric Robespierre! How's that, boys and girls?*

There's Drs. Berman and Ng socializing—a real bunch of yappy-de-yaps, don't ya think? And when I shuffle/drag my ass in, do these Chatty Cathys even take a breath and recognize my presence? Okay—they don't have to "Hail Caesar" me, but a *hello, howdy, how ya doing* would be nice—but noooo, *bupkis*, nothing, *nada, rien.*

I spot a nurse, and there's another lurking on the periphery, but I'm not interested in doing any optical gymnastics. Better to keep my field of vision narrow, continue to toe the line—the less I see, the better off I'll be. Unfortunately, as I approach the operating table, suspended right above (you'd have to be blind or, thankfully, drugged to miss it) is a huge light looking menacingly like . . . like a giant spacecraft hovering there, waiting to beam me up. The Zoladex mothership—nah . . .

I reach the table, and both the nurse and Dr. Kopman help me climb up, but to show them I'm no coward, I jump up (okay, maybe I'm exaggerating at bit), and then as the nurse straps my legs to the table, (where the hell does she think I'm going?), Dr. Kopman says, "I'm going to give you a little something to calm you down."

"I hope so, because I can hear the sound of my own heartbeat."

That's a joke, folks, but no one's laughing. I feel someone (probably The-Nurse-That-Lurks) putting tape on my eyes, and maybe I feel an IV being inserted. Then, I'm pretty sure Dr. Kopman's saying something about taking the express flight into oblivion . . . then—THEN I'M WAKING UP, natural as can be, as if the last few hours didn't exist. Without even the redeux of my ten-year-old tonsillectomy dream of a maniacal Mickey Mouse Thanksgiving Day Parade balloon descending in a swirl of black-and-red smoke, threatening to crush me like a pancake in front of my apartment building on West 74th Street.

Alive—I'm alive!—I'M FUCKING ALIVE! Colin Clive's in the house—this is all good—this is all very good. I take a moment to take inventory. My left hand's still hooked up to an IV bag with the contents half empty. I don't chance moving, but as far as I can tell nothing hurts; only I don't feel like celebrating because I'm shivering, chilled to the very bone. Gauzy, out-of-focus images wiggle in front of me, trying to shake themselves free and emerge out of the foggy whiteness that fills my line of vision, obscure as it is. Am I on an ice floe or the morgue room? Is that why it's glacier cold?

Marlowe's next to my bed, fingering the IV line with muscle-bound digits. I'd be more comfortable with a lion pawing at my throat, but you play the hand you're given.

"Listen, pally, quit your egg frying, it's all silk so far."

His eyes, now tiny twin points of steel grey in the cold fluorescent light of the recovery room, continue their staredown. I'm shaking like a leaf.

"Place is a freezer, but they'll be shoving you out in a couple, then piss in a cup and take it on the heel and toe."

"You really think I'm okay?"

"I said so, didn't I, pally?"

"Mr. Robespierre? Mr. Robespierre? I'm Janice—and you're in the main recovery area."

"I'm cold."

A face nods. "I'll bring you another blanket."

"Go with her," I tell Marlowe. "Make sure it's a warm one."

"Sure, pally, I'll take the air if you want."

I'm really shaking, worrying if it's a fever from an infection, or because they left something inside my prostate besides the seeds—like a sponge, scalpel or a

Mercedes S-Class? That's funny. A Mercedes. How they hell could they have gotten a vehicle through the narrow laparoscopic incisions, unless—UNLESS they lied, cut me from stem to Berman's summer home in the Hamptons (all doctors have summer homes in the Hamptons, don't you know?); that way they could certainly get a Mercedes into my prostate, no problemo. I'm lying absolutely motionless, don't want to rip open any holes—besides, the more inert I remain, the warmer I am, an important law of heat distribution I learned as a child who caught a mucous-filled, fever-and-chills cold at least once a month.

I feel gentle hands and a sudden draft as Recovery Nurse Janice lifts me up ever so slightly and fits an additional blanket around me.

"Here—is that better?"

"Ahh— thanks . . . " Is that even my voice, or one from another dimension?

"Are you feeling any pain?"

"No." I have no clue who's talking.

"I'm Janice. I'm the recovery nurse."

Shapes, then objects slowly come into focus. I see Recovery Nurse Janice. I nod. "I'm feeling jittery."

She smiles, pats my leg, and walks away.

Didn't you hear me? Janice! Janice! Where is she? JITTERY! JITTERY! NO ESCAPING THAT FOR ME! Gene's in the house and we're blinking furiously. Ouch! There's something in my left eye.

A sty? Damn—I know—chalazions—tiny pustules that develop when an oil gland in the eyelid becomes blocked—only I get'em when I'm anxious. Can you believe this shit! Even when you're unfucking conscious, these bastards can get to you. I'm blinking, rubbing—a no-no because a) it just makes it worse, and b) if you take that finger and rub the other eye you're going to infect them both.

Marlowe's now at the foot of my bed. "Hey pally . . . "

"Hey . . . " I close my eyes. Relax. *Thank you, God, for getting me through this. I really appreciate the fact I'm not dead, I have no pain, and I appear to be of clear mind.*

Be careful, Eric —don't go overboard and make promises you can't keep, like you're going to totally devote the rest of your life to helping the homeless find affordable housing.

I open my eyes. Marlowe's gone. I should have thanked Raymond Chandler when I was thanking God. I look around. I'm able to see clearly, although I definitely feel something in my left eye. I rub it. (Okay, I have no self-control.) I'm really feeling jittery. What's up with this? I lift my head slightly. There's Recovery Nurse Janice, talking on the phone. No one else around and nothing seriously scary nearby like a crash cart. She's off the phone.

"Nurse, Nurse!" My throat's dry, my voice weak and crackly. I clear my throat and take a deep breath. "Nurse, oh nurse!"

She turns. I clear my throat again because I'm feeling a lump in there. Recovery Nurse Janice approaches.

"Hi, I don't mean to bother you, but every time I blink, it feels like something's irritating my upper lid."

She bends over, examines the offending orb, gently pulling the lids up and down. I see Marlowe behind her, only he's strangely elongated, like his torso's being squeezed out of the toothpaste tube.

Recovery Nurse Janis pulls the upper lid up, then the lower down. "They're a little red, but I don't see anything. I'll get you a moist tissue and we'll see if that'll help. If it doesn't, I'll call the resident working in ophthalmology."

I feel her body heat and already I'm warming up. She smells of a flowery bouquet, maybe roses—not that I'm an expert. However, I am one on body heat, and wish Recovery Nurse Janice would stay until all my flesh is aflame—not going to happen.

I can't help myself; I'm rubbing my eye again. There, I think it's gone— nope, back again. One good thing: my eyesight's returned, and with it a lot more mental clarity. I have no pain, then again I've haven't moved an inch except for my left hand, which is at my eye again.

Whoa, look who's here—Dr. Kopman.

"Eric, how are you feeling?"

"Okay."

He feels my pulse. "Any pain?"

"My left eye, I think there's something in it."

He bends over, checks my eye. "It's a little red. It could be from the tape we put over your eyes."

"Why the tape?"

"Uh—well—things are always flying around the operating room. We also tape them shut to prevent the ducts from tearing, but we lubricate the eyes first, and that may be what's causing the discomfort. I'm going to get you an eyewash solution that will help. I'll be back in a minute."

Things flying around the OR, huh? I'm picturing Berman and Ng throwing scalpels at each other. *"No—I make the incisions!" "No, I'm more important—I put in the rads!"* How about when Ng opens the lead-lined container, it plays exploding popcorn machine, only instead of tasty kernels flying around, it's radioactive red-hots.

Back to reality—or what passes for it when you're thirty minutes out of surgery. Dr. Kopman bends over and applies a few drops of solution to my left eye.

"Let's see what this does."

No immediate relief. "Uh—could I keep that?"

"Well—I'm not supposed to but, here, tuck it away."

"Thanks."

"So, Eric—everything else all right—no pain anywhere?"

"I think I'm fine."

"Good."

"So when do they move me out of here?"

"They want to wait for the anesthetic to completely clear out, and that should be within the half-hour."

"Thank you, doctor."

"You're welcome."

My eye still hurts, but it's peculiar how this inconvenience is preoccupying my mind, not the operation or associated side effects, like the gram-negative bacteria found growing in hospitals and resistant to all antibiotics, with a kill ratio of one in four. How about radioactive seeds hotfooting it through my prostate, rendering me forever impotent? Let us not forget the fifteen percent possibility that cancer cells, too tiny to show up under the scrutiny of present-day analysis, have escaped into the general population, making this procedure null and void?

So—what's up with this eye fixation? Time to come clean—full disclosure and all that—as if you already didn't know: fixating on the inconsequential to deflect, deny, and bury the real threat is my coping mechanism—my MO for survival. As a child I was fixated on a fear of sleepwalking (only happened once) that shielded me from the psychic pain of insecurity—the kind that comes when your parents don't appear as well educated as those of your schoolmates. The second, and the one I'm experiencing today, first appeared the day I learned my mother had bone cancer, and continued off and on for two years until she passed and was thankfully released from her excruciatingly painful torment.

Recovery Nurse Janice leans over. "How are you?"

"Dr. Kopman came by, gave me something to soothe the irritation."

"Very good, because I paged the resident up in ophthalmology and he still hasn't returned my call. We should be moving you out shortly. We just have to wait for transport so they can take you back to Outpatient Recovery."

"Okay. I'm still feeling jittery, but not as bad."

She pulls away and gets ready to leave. Did she not get my cry for help? Does she not understand when I tell her I'm feeling jittery this is me saying, "GET ME A GODDAMN DOCTOR, I NEED FUCKING HELP!" What do I have to do to get help around here, bring Jack Torrance and his axe into the house? *Here's Johnny—smash, boom, smash, boom—scream!*

"Hey, pally, you don't want to take the bounce, do yah?"

"No. I want to stay."

"So be a wisehead." Marlowe's standing shoulder to shoulder with Recovery Nurse Janice, eyes growing more luminescent as they anticipate her next move; now stepping aside, allowing her room to pass, then resuming their customary staredown.

"My eye hurts, I'm cold all over, and still shaking like a leaf."

"Don't be a weak sister. Like I said, lie still until it's time to piss, then take it on the heel and toe."

"You really think I'm okay?"

"I'm putting you wise, ain't I, pally?"

I always liked Bogart as Marlowe—I mean, how can you beat his balls-to-the-wall performance in *The Big Sleep*?—but I loved Dick Powell as much in *Farewell, My Lovely*, which changed to *Murder, My Sweet,* because studio bigwigs didn't want audiences to think song-and-dance man Powell was making a musical. Powell's deadpan, laidback play and cagy hands-off approach was deadlier than Bogie's because it was unexpected; whoever saw a handsome dude talking the talk and walking the walk? Yet it is Bogart who's in the house, not Powell or Alan Ladd (another one of my favorite deadpan, dead-voice pretty boys) or the last actor you would expect, Mr. Fred MacMurray, who gives the ultimate gnarly noir performance in *Double Indemnity.*

"Yes, I killed him. I killed him for money—and a woman—and I didn't get the

money and I didn't get the woman. Pretty, isn't it?"

I feel better buoyed by these friendly and familiar characters, more real and supportive than perhaps is healthy—but then again am I less balanced than those who find solace in reading from the Apostles, characters some say are as imaginary as my silver-screen gumshoes? Hey—if Powell, Laddie, and Bogie played Peter, Paul, and Luke, I might be more of a churchgoer; I say, whatever floats your boat, as long as you don't try to capsize mine.

Marlowe turns. A hospital attendant pushing a gurney appears with Recovery Nurse Janis close on his heels. Marlowe winks, steps back, and out of the way. On the count of three, Nurse Janis and Hospital Attendant Guy, a black mountain disguised as a man, lift me gently off the bed and onto the gurney. I feel no pain.

The ceiling is rushing by: lights, air-conditioning ducts, partitions spider-webbed with dust. I want to make a joke, make this guy like me like a brother or at least a bro so he doesn't whip me into the wall like they do in roller derby.

How about this for a really, really bad dream? Wheel me down to the morgue, where bleary-eyed, overworked pathologists mistakenly slice me open, autopsy my live ass, discovering their fatal mistake when I gasp my last breath, too fucking late to do anything but cover me with a fucking sheet!

I'm through the doors and back in Ambulatory Surgery Unit Pre-Op (that now also passes for outpatient recovery). Man-Mountain Transport Guy and a nurse I've never seen before expertly lift me off the bed and very delicately ease me back onto my recliner, placing my rolling IV pole and bag to the left of me. Except for the IV in my hand, it's like I never left. Maybe I never did.

I gaze up to my right and there's my black clothing bag hanging on the cubicle wall. I remember: they park it someplace safe, then return it.

New Nurse smiles as Man-Mountain Transport Guy pushes the gurney out into the hall and out of view. "How are you feeling, Mr. Robespierre?" she asks.

"Okay . . . "

"Sit for a while. If you need to go to the bathroom, it's right over there."

"Okay . . . "

"Is there anyone waiting for you in the visitors' lounge?"

"Uh-huh—my daughter."

"I'll call over there."

"Her name's Gillian—Gillian Robespierre."

I notice the nametag—*Maureen*, but for some unexplained reason don't give her figure a second look and instead look straight into her eyes. "Thank you, Maureen."

She smiles.

My affected orb is smarting, but thankfully not so bad that I have to rub it. I move ever so gently to my right—not wanting to tear the IV out of my hand—reach up, and open the clothing bag. My wallet, keys, and cell phone are right where I left them.

The outer doors keep opening and closing—but no Gillian. I dial her number.

"Hi, honey. Yep, I'm okay. You can come in now. Where are you? You're kidding! Well—just come in."

A moment later my darling daughter appears.

"Boy, am I happy to see you," I say.

She's smiling and appears relieved, but I also see she's a little apprehensive and tired—very tired. Getting up at five-thirty in the morning will do that to you, compounded by the anxiety of the event, which drains her face, deepens the purplish-black rings under her beautifully rounded big brown eyes, now even more pronounced against the blanched whiteness of her skin.

She bends down. I lean up to meet her. We hug. A nice, warm, gentle hug, maybe too gentle, too tentative.

"I'm okay. I won't break."

She squeezes me tighter. I feel her tote bag brush against my back. She gently releases me and I sit back down.

"I'm thirsty. I guess I can drink, what do you think?"

She shrugs. I point to the nurses' station.

"Why don't you ask? In the meantime, I'm going to see if I can pee." I lift myself up. I'm not feeling dizzy. My legs aren't wobbly.

"You need help, pally?" Marlowe stands in front of me.

"Thanks, but I think I can make it."

He moves out of the way. I take a few cautious steps, careful to bring the rolling IV pole with me. The hallway's not spinning, my legs still haven't turned to jelly. I'm doing okay. Marlowe's next to me, moving with me, step by step, ready to catch me if I take a header.

"Nice and easy does it, pally."

We pause in front of the bathroom.

"You don't mind if I wait outside, do you?" He grins. I nod.

"Not for nothing, but you got yourself a fine young daughter."

I see that, Marlowe—and thanks.

I pull open the bathroom door, then close it gently behind me. I look in the mirror—pale, but not as deathly white as my daughter. I carefully lift up my hospital gown, gently grab my very limp penis, and hope for the best.

"If you cannot pass urine after the procedure, a catheter is placed into the bladder and is removed one to two days later."

I fear the insertion. I fear the pain. I remember, as if it were yesterday and not twenty years ago, that awful day I take my father to see his urologist. He's in the early stages of treatment that will successfully prolong his life, however, that day looked like his last. My father is a large, friendly man who never exhibits any toughness, but is one of the strongest men I've ever met and who, well into his eighties, can still lift me up and toss me to one side without breaking a sweat or stride. It's only in his last two years of life I see his strength slightly diminish, but never his tolerance for pain, right up until the horrible end when we have to give him morphine to stop his fussing and fidgeting. There are no outward signs he is in any discomfort, which any ordinary mortal would experience as screaming agony.

So you can imagine how unusual it is on the day in question when after this particular exam my father doesn't spend his customary time flirting with the receptionist. I normally don't like to interrupt Father Casanova when he's making his moves, so I wait in my seat, finally getting up when I see him slowly shuffling toward me, the overhead fluorescents illuminating his dead-pale face. He reaches out to me when I get to him and try to assist him to the door (picture Harry Potter aiding Rubeus Hagrid). In the cab I ask how it went, and he stoically mumbles something unintelligible. When I press him further, ask if it was painful (how stupid and insensitive was that?), he grimaces, nods, and simply says, "They stuck something up my pee-pee."

"They stuck something up my pee-pee." No matter how childishly expressed, his words fill me with dread. It is at that moment I vow nobody will ever stick anything up my pee-pee—no way—no how.

My father's sweet smile fades and I'm face to face with my own reflection in the shiny silver towel dispenser. I stare down into the bowl—not even the tiniest drop, nor the slightest urge to douse the porcelain. My bladder's totally empty, that's why. Right? Right!

I flush out of habit, wash my hands and open the door, careful to maneuver the IV pole, watchful not to tear out my tethered connection and bleed out on the hallway floor. Marlowe is still there and I see Gillian behind him. I try to put on a happy face.

"I guess I need to drink some water?"

Gillian nods, smiles; thankfully, she can't read my mind. I slowly approach my cubicle and ease myself down onto the recliner. No pain, no dizziness, no headache, and my eye doesn't hurt anymore, either. Only I can't pee—and I can't go home.

Gillian has brought Nurse Maureen to my cubicle. "It's okay to drink," Maureen says. She points to a six-ounce bottle on the table next to my recliner that must have been placed there while I was in the OR. I quickly drain it.

"Would you like more?"

"Yes, please."

"There is also fruit juice, orange, apple, cranberry, or V8—and soda, diet and regular, Coke, and ginger ale."

I look at Gillian.

"I'll take a cranberry," Gillian answers.

"Could I have some water and an apple juice?" I whisper hoarsely.

"Absolutely. I'll be back in a moment to take your BP," smiles Maureen.

Gillian wants to know how it went, and I have to admit it wasn't bad. I start to give her a blow by blow. Marlowe moves in next to her, but when I see him shaking his head in disapproval, I nod and cut to the chase.

"I went into the OR, the anesthesiologist gave me a shot, and the next thing I know I'm waking up, it's freezing cold, but I have no pain or soreness, only a minor eye irritation and the shakes, which I now remember the recovery nurse saying were due to the after effects of the anesthetic."

Marlowe cracks the tiniest of smiles.

Attached to my partition wall is a magazine rack. Gillian takes a look, but nothing interests her.

"Why don't you look in the other rooms, maybe you'll find something there?" I suggest.

She wanders off. I decide to make a few calls. I see I have four voice mails. Before I have a chance to retrieve my messages, Gillian returns with a couple of magazines.

"I found these next door."

"Great."

"You want something to read?"

"Maybe later. I think I'll call Nick."

"I spoke with him while you were in surgery. He wanted me to call him as soon as I heard anything."

I call him. I blame technology for no longer having to memorize phone numbers, but as I scroll down the list of contacts, I have a pang of guilt this laziness that extends to my own kids.

Nick is happy to hear my voice, almost as happy as I am to hear his, but I'm not going to cry or get overly dramatic.

"Things are good. The surgery went fine, I have no pain and I'm just waiting to pee so I can get the hell out of Dodge."

Gillian's listening, hanging on every word, looking for signs of untruths, but I'm careful not to show any catheter concerns. *"Fear is the mind-killer, fear is the mind-killer . . ."*

I tell Nick how happy I am that Gilly's here, how she met me at 6:00 a.m., how we got to the hospital an hour early, how she's been a rock and how happy I am she's here with me now. Gillian turns red and pretends to read her magazine. I suddenly feel that by complimenting Gillian I may be slighting Nick, maybe even giving him a guilty feeling for not being here with me, so I take great pains to make sure he again knows I'm okay with his situation, that it was my strong wish he not cancel out on his shoot, forcing the production company to hire another cinematographer and costing Nick a large paycheck and perhaps the loss of future freelance with that company.

"Get back to work. Call me later, or I'll try you when I get home. Okay?"

"Okay. I love you, Pop."

"I love you, too, and I can't tell you how much I appreciate the love and concern you've shown me these last few months. You're a great son, all I could hope for."

"Thanks, Pop."

Gillian is smiling.

Nurse Maureen is back with three bottles of water, two small cans of cranberry and apple juice, a couple of chocolate cupcakes, straws, and little plastic cups. She looks up and sees that the IV bag is empty.

"I'm going to take your BP, then detach the IV bag, but it's hospital procedure to leave the IV in until you're ready to leave the hospital."

"Sure—not a problem." I take a few deep breaths. *"Fear is the mind-killer, fear is the mind-killer."* It works. I'm able to keep the pressure down enough to satisfy Nurse Maureen. She carefully detaches the IV; what a pro, I don't feel a thing. (Naturally, I'm not looking.) I'm smiling at Gillian, who is smiling back, but, unlike me, unable to keep her eyes off of Nurse Maureen.

Next thing I know, Nurse Maureen's wheeling away the IV pole, smiling, telling us to just walk over to the nurses' station if we need her and notify her the minute I urinate so she can get the discharge papers ready.

"Absolutely, you got it—not a problem."

I'm screwed. Marlowe comes up behind Gillian and gives me a dirty look.

"What—you think I'll be able to pee?"

Marlowe stays silent, his unblinking grey eyes, boring into mine, seem to be speckled with red flares, so bright I have to turn away. Gillian pours herself some cranberry juice, offers me some.

"I'm going with the apple," I say. I pour the contents into a plastic cup. Before my radiation I'm a short sips guy, now I'm able to empty a cup in a single gulp. *It's a bird, it's a plane, it's Super Swallower!* I gobble down the chocolate cupcake in three bites (some things don't change), then it's time to empty a second bottle of water.

A new nurse, Nurse Anne, appears.

"Hi, Mr. Robespierre."

"Hi."

"Everything all right?"

"Yep."

"Have you gone to the bathroom yet?"

"Nope."

She smiles indulgently. "Let me know as soon as you do, and then you can be discharged."

I nod. I'm thinking Damocles, only it isn't a sword and it's a different "head" that's going to be screwed with.

"What's the joke? . . . Why does a man's penis have a hole in it? So oxygen can get to his brain. Ha, ha, ha . . . ."

Marlowe just stares, his square jawline hardening in disgust.

Laugh, and the whole world laughs with you—not today, boyo.

ROUND 33

To summarize: I couldn't pee, they inserted the Foley (short for *Foley catheter*), showed me how to change the sterile drainage bags (500-ml. leg bag to 2-liter bed bag), I went home, couldn't change the bags, developed clots, couldn't pee, rushed to doctor, had Foley flushed, continued to bleed, kept Foley, urine cleared, went to Berman, removed Foley.

Talk about going into the *pissoire* . . .

From what I read on the Internet, less than three percent of patients who undergo seed implantation have to go home with a Foley. There are no statistics on how many patients jerry-rig Foleys to trash bags and sleep sitting up for four straight nights.

Talk about going into the *pissoire* . . .

Dr. Berman is his gentle self, and I only give off one *whoa* and a wince—or is it a wince and a *whoa*?—when he deflates the Foley balloon and expertly pulls out the tubing. Free at last—Mr. Floppy's free at last!

I have to stick around the office for another half-hour to make sure I can pee and my urine is clear. My urine's been clear for the last twelve hours, so I'm confident on that score, but whether or not I can pee without the Foley is another matter.

"So, pally, what's the score?"

Marlowe's been in the waiting room the entire time, reading the latest car and sports magazines, and when I give the shamus the thumbs up, he casually pockets a *Road & Track*, puts on his coat (he has never removed his hat as long as I have known him), and heads for the door.

I think about walking home, but not having slept for more than an hour at a time since Sunday convinces me that when I get to 14th Street, I should take a bus across town. I do make one concession. I stop at Circuit City to look at the HD sets. I think I should splurge and treat myself—I deserve it. I faced my biggest fear and lived to tell about it—and now I think I should tell about it . . . so let's go back four days. Right? Right!

Talk about going into the *pissoire* . . .

Hospital procedure calls for the insertion of the Foley catheter into the bladder when it becomes obvious the patient still cannot pee on his own. Nurse Maureen and I conspire to prolong the inevitable for more than an hour, until Dr. Berman orders otherwise.

Aided by a shift change, I have been successful in my delaying tactics, but no matter how much I drink, bathe Mr. Floppy in hot water, or walk up and down the corridor, I cannot urinate. What I don't know, and what causes Dr. Berman displeasure (I use the term loosely), is the harm I could be doing to my bladder. When it becomes a choice between an exploding blue balloon or the dreaded insertion, I realize there's no choice. I'm alarmed when another Man-Mountain Transport Guy wheels in a gurney and I'm told to lie absolutely still. Nurse Margaret (Nurse Maureen's able-bodied replacement and the last of my lassie ladies) asks Gillian to wait outside. My daughter can't wait to get out, and I don't blame her. Why should she have to see her father like this? I only hope her mother and I have the good sense to sneak onto an ice floe and float away before she or my son face life's ultimate calamity.

Nurse Margaret closes the curtain, and I finally face the inevitable. Even Marlowe backs up until he brushes against my clothing bag. I grip the sides of the gurney.

"Will it hurt much?"

How insane am I? As if she is going to tell me the truth!

"Just a little discomfort. I've been doing this for over thirty years—so just relax."

"Fear is the mind-killer . . . fear is the mind-killer . . ." Why in the world my eyes aren't closed is the sixty-four-thousand-dollar question, but they aren't, so I'm treated to the sight of the unfurling of the Anaconda. Oh yeah, this is no thin-tubing motherfucker—and I tell them so. (Meekly)

"Is it possible to put me out?"

(Pause) "Oh, we don't do that."

(Even more pathetically) "How about a local?"

(Another pause) "You won't need that—it'll be over in a minute."

"Fear is the mind-killer . . . fear is the mind-killer . . ." My eyes are closed almost as tightly as my grip on the gurney or my sphincter that's going into spasm thinking I've lost my mind and signed up for Palates.

"The truth—I don't think you can handle the truth!" Oh, Jack, yes, they can.

A sterilizing agent is applied to the tip of the penis. The Foley catheter is inserted and gently pushed into the urethra. When it reaches the bladder, its tiny tip is inflated with sterile water to create a balloon, which keeps the Foley in place and prevents it from slipping out of the bladder.

How does the fucking truth feel? A little pressure, some discomfort and then a few stabs of pain—and then, a *whoosh* and my bladder begins to sing the "Hallelujah Chorus."

"See—I told you so. Didn't I, pally?"

"Yeah—well—then why do you look white as a sheet?"

Marlowe doesn't answer. Thank God, he doesn't or I would have taken a swing at the big galoot.

The ugly, brownish-yellow tube is fastened to Mr. Floppy by thin strips of white tape, and I feel so sorry for the little fella, who looks like he tried to roll himself up into my groin, but got caught three-quarters of the way in.

Nurse Margaret and Man-Mountain Transport Guy carefully help me off the gurney and back into the recliner. No real pain, but definitely a strange feeling of pressure and just a pinprick when the tubing pulls at the tip. Poor Mr. Floppy. The Foley is connected to a large plastic container bag Nurse Margaret carefully attaches to the side of the recliner.

"I'm going to send you home with a smaller leg bag that fastens to your thigh so you can walk around more easily. I'm also going to show you how to take that off, and switch it for the one you have on now that's big enough to collect all your nighttime urine and will enable you to sleep through."

"Thank you."

"I'm going to call your daughter in—is that all right?"

"Sure—fine—no problem."

I make sure I'm covered up. I reach for a bottle of orange juice and take a huge gulp.

Successfully putting on one's jeans (*sans* Fruit of The Loom) without touching the tubing and clearing an ever-inflating thigh must be done with extreme care; however, if you emulate Clint Eastwood strapping on his gigantor Spaghetti Western six-shooter, it's a piece of linguini. Walking with this monstrous weapon, and then babysitting it in the back of a New York City cab (yeah—we told him to go slow and avoid the potholes—so what's your point?) is another matter.

As soon as I get home, I change into an extra-large and loose-fitting nightshirt (my father's), and figure out if I put a soft pillow under my *tush* and just sit quietly, my rectum won't feel quite so sore. I'm relived the operation (okay—

procedure) is over and I'm finally home again, but I still feel oddly unhinged, as if none of this is really happening and I'm in some kind of dreamlike state.

Dum dee dum dum.

I call Nick, Helen, Ellyn, and Ira, but I'm so worn out I don't have the energy to rehash all the day's events, so I'm brief and always upbeat. While I make my calls, Gillian orders comfort food from my favorite Thai restaurant. I've got two pages of instructions laying out my post-op drug regimen, and I'm paying strict attention to what to take and when and how many. The food comes and my appetite is surprisingly good.

I'm beginning to feel better than I expect, considering the snake snaking out of my snake and the baggie uncomfortably strapped to my thigh, its contents sloshing like ground glass in a blender every time I move. Oh—I'm over the nasty part, (don't have trouble emptying the thing, and do it with regularity), however, there's blood in my urine, therefore, the less I visit the bathroom, the happier I am.

If you cannot pass urine after the procedure, a catheter is placed into the bladder and is removed one to two days later. It is normal to have some blood in the urine, which will drain from the catheter. If it becomes severe and/or is associated with large blood clots, call your urologist.

So, beside being in shock and scared to death of peeing blood, I'm not really concerned when, just before Gillian leaves (I decide I'll be okay by myself), we change bags. Remember—in the hospital I'm watching Nurse Margaret and I know Gillian's also paying close attention when she demonstrates how to change the bag, however—HOWEVER—I don't care if you can field strip this thing blindfolded in the ER while hemorrhaging—WHEN YOU GET HOME, YOU WILL FUCK IT UP!

Try as we might, for the next thirty minutes, Gillian and I cannot unfasten the little bag without yanking the tubing so hard it threatens to break, or worse, pull the entire Foley out (don't even picture that!).

We read the instructions that come with the bag, even go onto the Internet and look at instructions there. Gillian tries it. I try it. We both try it together. We are calm, cool, and collected. I take precautions to empty the bag before we start and manage to hold off urinating, because there is something profoundly disturbing about watching your bodily fluids bubbling up in a baggie.

I send Gillian home. There's no sense to her staying. We embrace and both of us are crying. It has been a long and exhausting day, but it's over, and thankfully everything is okay.

"I love you, sweetheart. You're a father's dream come true—my darling, darling daughter."

"I love ya, Pops . . . "

I have two bed bags, so I can afford to snip off the tubing on one and attempt to attach it to the spigot of my leg bag. A keener eye would realize the diameters didn't match and no amount of taping could possibly work. I try to lie down, but unless my leg is perpendicular to the floor, gravity will not allow the urine to flow through the Foley, resulting in a reverse flow of urine back into the bladder if not corrected. This "back up into the bladder" business is something Dr. Berman warned me about in the hospital and something I now take very, very seriously. I carefully remove my leg bag and attach it to the side of the bed, but the tubing is too short and it tugs painfully at my penis.

When all appears lost, the answer comes to me, and with that answer, an awareness that out of this crisis is revealed my life's purpose.

Can I have an amen? AMEN!

You see, my brothers, that evening—just as God hands Moses The Ten Commandments—He puts a giant trash bag into my hands, and I know if I open Foley bag into my magical gift and hang the sucker at the right downward angle, I can turn five hundred milliliters into thirty gallons (fish into loaves comes into my mind along with the Mosses analogy) and find a way to lay my head down on a pillow and sleep.

Can I have an amen? AMEN!

This is my epiphany, this is my purpose, to tell you, my brothers—make sure you have a full box of giant trash bags, white ones, so you can see the color of your urine, and tape— not Scotch Tape, but strong stuff like gaffer's tape, because you don't want that heavy bag collapsing and spilling out all over the floor.

Can I have an amen? AMEN!

Now—had I remembered the story of Jesus, I would have realized finding one's purpose don't mean a thing unless you get that zing back in your thang.

Tuesday starts off with me still throwing clots and even though it's off and on, (one minute I'm passing clumps and it's Red River, the next a drop or two and the Big Muddy), Mr. Floppy definitely don't have no zing, and I'm really feeling for the little fella. But on Tuesday evening things *really* go south. There's tightness when I try to go, and I immediately realize a clot must be stuck up in the tubing, and until I can pass it, I won't be able to urinate. I drink. I wrap poor Mr. Floppy in a hot towel (careful to avoid the tip), but when Wednesday morning comes and I still can't pee, I know there is big, big trouble in River City. True, I'm not feeling any pain, but I know it can come at any minute. I remember Lou telling me about his blockage and how it made him double over in pain, and if this image isn't enough to scare the living daylights out of me, there's the old "back up into the bladder" to deal with.

I call the hospital and try to get a hold of Nurse Maureen or Nurse Margaret. I get someone else from their station, but I just can't come by and have a nurse fix the problem; I need to go to the emergency room. I dress, grab a cab, and head toward the hospital. It's no fun leaving the comfort of my couch knowing any movement can exacerbate the already raw penis, even though I have been diligently putting Neosporin on the affected area to prevent it from getting worse, as well as, to prevent infection. Miraculously, still no pain, not even the slightest bladder discomfort. I can make it— *"Fear is the mind-killer, fear is the mind-killer."* Thank God Marlowe's in the cab with me, only I can't stop him muttering about taking a shot at the deodorant, shaped like a silver crown, that sits atop the dashboard.

"Please, make sure you don't hit a pothole—I have many stitches!"

I'm yelling because the guy's talking nonstop on his cell in Farsi or some Indian or Pakistani dialect when suddenly it dawns on me, *Call Dr. Berman—get him to contact the ER so I can be seen quickly and by somebody special.*

I reach his service, leave a message and a minute later I get a call back. Dr. Berman says to go to his office and Dr. Stein will take care of me. Halleluiah! Halleluiah! We are halfway across town when I tell the cabbie to change directions and head down to 9th Street between Broadway and Irving Place. For some reason, maybe because he's seen Marlowe's threatening .45 in his rearview, Farsi Cabby has reduced his speed, and when he follows my instructions and makes a left and catches the light at Fifth and 19th Street, it's a smooth-as-silk turn. Why I didn't think to call Dr. Berman in the first place is beyond me, but you can be sure I'm not going to make that mistake again.

There's no one in the waiting room when I arrive and only a lone receptionist at the desk—then again, it's 7:45 a.m., and the office doesn't officially open until 8:00 a.m.

Marlowe doesn't even have time to find a magazine before Dr. Mark Stein appears.

"Eric?"

I stand, careful not to juggle my six-shooter or tug at Mr. Floppy. "Yep!"

I follow him into my home away from home. This is where Dr. Berman gave me my biopsy.

"So, you're having trouble urinating?"

"I think the Foley's clogged."

"Let's have a look. You don't need to remove your jeans, just pull them down and then your shorts." He's flipping through my file, scanning Dr. Berman's voluminous notes. "I see you had your implants on Monday. How did that go?"

"Actually, pretty good. No pain, just this damn catheter."

Dr. Stein begins to examine the catheter. "Dr. Ang did your implants?"

"He was great. Everyone was great. Dr.—uh—I can't remember the name of the anesthesiologist—whoa!"

"Sorry, did that hurt?"

"Just a little tug."

"I'm just going to flush it out."

"You mean, you don't have to remove it?"

"No, just a little saline solution." I see him shoot a syringe full of saline into the Foley through feeder line.

"Oh—so that's what that's for?"

Now I remember, Nurse Maureen used that opening to fill up the balloon. Why did I say Nurse Maureen, when it was Nurse Margaret who took care of the Foley?

"There—all done."

I see the drainage bag quickly filling up. "I'm still throwing clots. Dr. Berman said it would be a week?"

Dr. Stein doesn't choose to ease my anxiety, or perhaps he just doesn't see Berman's notation: *TREAT THIS PATIENT WITH CARE–HE'S A FRAIDY CAT!* "You can get dressed now. I advise you empty the bag before you leave. It'll be easier walking that way."

I am so relieved I begin a nonstop monologue that turns into a stand-up bit in which I describe, in all its magical glory, my trash-bag epiphany. I especially think my reenactment of Moses getting the tablets (substituting garbage bag for the tablets) is particularly hilarious. Although Dr. Stein doesn't look at me while I'm doing my performance (he's busy updating my file into the computer), he does crack a grin or two. Unfortunately, Dr. Stein doesn't have any leg bags, only the larger size versions, otherwise, he would be glad to change my bag. I'm disappointed, but I understand.

Dr. Berman (himself) calls me that afternoon (I told you he's a god), and assuming my urine stays clear for two days running, asks me to come in on Friday (today) for the removal of my trusty Italian six-shooter. I go through a trash bag a day and almost half a roll of gaffer's tape, managing twenty minutes of sleep here and there, slumped at a ninety-degree angle at the side of the couch, propped up against a mound of bed pillows (sitting on one as well) in my father's nightshirt, still eating take-out from my Thai place (Grandma's Chicken Noodle keeps me alive) and feeling very pasha-like one minute and eunuch-in-palace the next—but there's no more blockage and clots. My urine finally clears.

So—there's the long and the short of it, which brings us full circle!

Circuit City really knows how to display their HD TVs in the best possible way, and I'm torn between watching *Pirates of the Caribbean: At World's End* or yesterday's Yankee 2–1 victory over the Padres. I have to stop myself from shuffling between the two like I still have a baggie full of pee attached to my right thigh.

Come on, brain, forget it—and while you're at it, erase those images of me dragging trash bags loaded with nighttime urine to the bathroom, emptying them and watching the bowl turn blood-red.

"Excuse me, can you tell me the difference between this Sony and the Samsung?"

ROUND 34

CALL me crazy, but I miss coming to this place. Oh—don't get me wrong, I'm no addict. I can stop taking radiation anytime I want. *Prove it!* I've been off it for two months! How come I come by every week? I like the feta cheese over at the Chelsea Dinner . . .

Post-partum-radiation-in-the-cranium migraine.

The hugs keep coming. Tight, affectionate wrap-arounds that grab my heartstrings and don't let go.

"You look great, Eric."

"Look at that tan!"

"So, you've finally come back to see us, huh?"

"You look terrific! How are you feeling?"

Barbara checks my records in the computer. "You have to go to registration."

"Yep, I figured they want to see if my insurance is up to date."

It seems like yesterday that I'm sitting and waiting to go in for a treatment and then see a guy come in for his follow-up scan, have his records checked by Barbara on the computer, and then get sent off to Registration to get the proper authorization. I envied those guys and tried to send my body into theirs so I could be over and done with my treatment. It's hard to believe my time has come.

My insurance info checks out, and I'm back, waiting only a few minutes when a therapist calls my name and leads me into a small, unfamiliar room down the corridor from Mr. Linear Accelerator 1.

"Hi, you look well."

"Thanks, you do, too."

"Take care."

"You, too."

More friendly faces: nurses, therapists, but no hugs—too busy rushing patients into treatment rooms.

Well, hello, Mr. Donut. The open MRI machine dominates the narrow room. To my left: a shelf, a window above it looking out into the corridor, then a wall and a closed cabinet. On the opposite side, all sorts of portable monitors and a table filled with medical instruments. The rest of the room is all Mr. Donut. The therapist opens my file and looks at my photo, then me, then back at the photo.

"It's not my best angle. I'd be willing to pay for more photos," I quip.

He laughs.

"Nine, thirty, forty-two." I volunteer the info, then realize a phony could read it off the chart. *Yeah—like there are people who want to steal your MRI time. Please Eric, get psychiatric help before it's too late.*

"Mr. Robespierre, would you remove all metal objects?"

"Do I have to get undressed?"

"No, sir. Just take off your shoes."

"How long will it last?"

"About five minutes. We're just taking pictures of your lower abdomen to see if everything is back to normal."

He's smiling as if he thinks I don't know the real fucking reason I'm here—like maybe my organs changed shape, moved to other parts of my body, someone else's—or vanished completely

It takes more time to remove all my metal objects than to go through the MRI, nevertheless, when I leave, my hands are shaking and my legs feel that familiar Goodyear Tire feeling.

"Have some coffee, a health bar."

"How is your summer going? I bet you're a Hamptons guy?"

"Do you still see Lou?"

"You really look good. So—tell us everything."

Connie, Elizabeth, Barbara, Pauline—the entire gang is here and they surround me. I feel truly cared for, and think of how best to answer their questions.

During the night I get up every two hours to pee. The funny part about urgency issues is it takes a second or two before it comes out, a little tightness, some discomfort, but compared to having the Foley, no biggie. Flomax helps, and if I take Aleve I last three hours; no blood in my urine or stool and the soreness in my rectum is almost gone, but if I'm sitting for a long time it hurts a little unless I'm sitting on something soft. I just had the MRI, so I don't know if my prostate is where it's supposed to be, but since everybody tells me I look good, I guess my stuff's where it's supposed to be. Oh, one more thing— MR. FLOPPY IS DEAD MEAT AND I FEEL LIKE A FUCKING EUNUCH!

"I feel fine, ladies — thank you for asking . . . ."

Everybody is smiling—we all must have slept with hangers in our mouths.

"Don't be a stranger. You know where we are."

"I love the music you made for me."

"Thanks for the *Yummy Hunter's Guide*—I really love it!"

"Me, too!"

"Take a health bar or some fruit with you."

"Bye!"

"Bye!"

I really miss this place. Out in the hall, I wipe away a tear. A patient passes me as she heads toward Radiation. She forces a sad smile. She thinks I'm dying, when really I'm just beginning to feel alive again.

Round 35

THE office is nearly empty; there are only two young guys—hip, early thirties—and an unshaven, unkempt geezer in his seventies. Wonderful! I go directly to the front desk and recognize the Hispanic receptionist who greets me enthusiastically.

"Hello—Eric!"

"I'm early."

"We like early. Just sign in."

I'm the last scheduled appointment. I sign next to my printed name. We exchange further pleasantries. I feel very much at home here, so much so that I put my fleece shell under my coat and hang them right up on the rack, empty except for one other coat, hanging four hangers away.

Don't get too comfy—today is Have-Your-Prostate-Manually-Fucked-With Day. Suppose the exam uncovers problems in River City or the bloodletting reveals an increased PSA—what then, brave boy?

"Screw it, pally."

I didn't see Marlowe come in.

"Yeah—screw it, pally."

The two thirty-somethings are called in. Strange—they're not sitting together. I see them greeted by Lovely Blonde Nightingale. I smile, but she doesn't even notice me. How quickly they forget. The two guys go into different examining rooms. Okay, they aren't together. Okay, they aren't lovers having a spat and here for an STD exam so they can play the blame game.

I open my Soho Apple-store bag, pull out the Ian Rankin book, and for a sec look at the three HDMI cables. *Jesus Christ on a Popsicle stick, I'm actually spending over two grand on an HDTV and digital camera!* I'm suddenly swept up in my usual spend/don't spend-live/don't live soap opera. There's a precipitous drop in the you-can't-take-it with-you chemical neurotransmitter—the tight-ass-Scrooge chems are taking over. *Hold it, Masked Man! It's Manually-Fuck-Up-Your-Prostate Day! Get with the* carpe diem, *pally. Right? Right!*

I open the Rankin book. It occurs to me that from day one of this prostate business, this wonderful mystery writer has brightened my day. I've read at least two dozen books by various authors during this journey, but it always seems whenever I'm visiting a doctor or having a treatment it's a Rankin book by my side. Today, it's *Naming of the Dead*, a terrific read, not withstanding the unfriendly-to-cancer-patient title.

I know I'm now in a comfy spot, because I'm able to concentrate and read a couple of pages, but that all changes when I hear Yiddish, the secret language of my parents, coming from the direction of The Unshaven One. I swear it sounds like he's praying. Okay—I'm okay with that as long as he's not saying the Prayer for the Dead and looking in my direction. I'm just staring at the page now, maybe going on a minute, the words completely out of focus. No way I can concentrate when I hear one of the gay-or-not-gay men come out from the reception area, pass me and leave, giving me the opportunity to sneak a peek at The Unshaven One, who doesn't seem to be moving his lips, either in prayer or cell-phone chatter. Only one conclusion: he's mumbling to himself, and I'm alone in the waiting room with a nut job. No, I'm not. Marlowe's got my back.

"You got that right, pally."

Lovely Blonde Nightingale appears. "Irving, Eric—come with me."

Irving is quick on his feet, and by the time I take my glasses off and stick my hardcover back into my Apple bag, he's standing next to me.

"It's the dance team of Irving and Eric, together again."

Lovely Blonde Nightingale smiles at my little quip, but my eyes don't hold hers and I know for certain she doesn't remember me.

"You're Irving, too?"

Irving must be a little deaf or completely out of his mind.

"No—I'm Eric."

Irving nods, but I'm not sure anyone knows why.

Lovely Blonde Nightingale points me into the first examining room to my right. I enter. Ahh—returning to the scene of the pain, are we? I turn. I'm alone in the room. I take off my sweatshirt, put it on the back of the metal chair, pull the chair away from the window, sit, put on my glasses, take out my book, remember I need to give a urine sample, go into the hall and spot Lovely Blonde Nightingale.

"Do you want a sample?" I ask her.

"Yes."

"Which bathroom should I use?"

"The one behind you."

She points—more like a wave. This part of the office is a warren of examining rooms, storerooms, and bathrooms, and I'm lost, confused by my confusion, because back in the day I knew my way around this place. Ha—back in the day—the scene of the pain when it's hormone shots, biopsies, and test results—definitely moments unmusical.

I approach the far door, see it's a treatment room, then turn into a corridor, to the right a bathroom. I try the door—locked. Okay, I'm going into the waiting-room area, where I know there's another bathroom. I head back, spot Lovely Blonde Nightingale, and tell her what I'm doing so she doesn't think I'm running out on them.

"Don't forget to bring the sample back out here."

I nod. I know the drill.

Oh, I'm so smart. The bathroom is free and I see plenty of empty vials. I have no trouble providing a sample. Long gone are those nervous days of yesteryear when "Pee now" meant holding my piece forever. Now all I have to do is look at a urinal and my vial runneth over—one of the perks of prostate cancer, the medicos forget to tell you. There is one tiny problem.

"I can't find a pen," I tell the receptionist.

"Here—take this and leave it in the bathroom—I've got plenty."

"Sure, thanks."

I calmly return to the bathroom, my full-up held at my side and out of sight. The face in the mirror is a far cry from the one who once became unnerved when he had to write *Eric Robespierre* along the tiny wrap-around label affixed to an easily crushed little plastic vial filled with hot piss.

Damn, Boyo—you're actually smiling!

ROUND 36

OKAY, time to stop putting off the inevitable and call Dr. Berman for my test results. I really don't think there's a problem, because if there were he would have called me immediately. I get right through to the office, then get put on hold and after a moment or two—I'm disconnected. This is a first, and if I weren't the poster boy for mental-health week, I'd be thinking they don't want to talk to me, because who in their right mind wants to tell you you're dying? I'm dialing again, explain my problem, get transferred to a nurse who looks up my chart.

"PSA minus zero-point-one, urine culture normal, urine analysis normal, testosterone test still not back but results should be coming in today. Would you like Dr. Berman to call you?"

I'm furiously writing everything down. "Yes."

"What number?"

I give her the number, then ask, "Okay—what's the difference between a urine culture and urine analysis?"

"A urine culture tests for an infection and the urine analysis—you know, I'm not sure — let me put you on with a nurse. . . . "

"Hi, this is Diane."

She sounds like Lovely Blonde Nightingale.

"Hi, I know who you are. This is Eric Robespierre."

"Hi." Diane explains: "Urine culture tests to see if there are bacteria in the urine, urine analysis tests for red and white blood cells."

I'm thinking I'm hearing a Spanish accent, and that's not Lovely Blonde Nightingale. I'd like to play detective and figure it out, but I can't without losing concentration and already I feel my powers fading. I have another concern, and I might as well come out with it now that I know it's not the love of my fantasy life.

"I guess the testosterone test is for testosterone?"

"Yes. We want to see if you have too much or too little—then there's a problem."

"So—when those results come in, Dr. Berman will call me?"

"Yes—that's right."

"Okay. Thanks, and take care."

"You, too."

Too much or too little, then there's a problem. What the hell does that mean? I can always look it up on the Internet. *Oh, no. Those worms will stay in the can.* I walk away from the computer, return to the bedroom, and put the phone back onto its base. I stare at the laundry that's just come out of the dryer: half the stuff is folded, the other half strewn across the bed, a job unfinished—one I interrupted when I decided to stop procrastinating and call Dr. Berman.

Okay—I made the call, so now let's fold. No—another cup of coffee and some music: *The Pearl Fishers*, Bizet's magical opera, full of great tunes and gorgeous arias, especially the friendship duet *"Au Fond du Temple Saint"*—guaranteed to send happy brain chemicals cascading over my neurons, sparking them into electrical ecstasy. Oh—if only the music could send the Big T into Mr. Floppy.

No more than ten minutes pass when the phone rings. The caller ID says Dr. Berman's office and I know it'll be the doc and not someone saying, "Hold on for Dr. Berman." I quickly head into the living room, where my pad and pen sit next to my computer.

"Eric—Dr. Berman."

"Hi."

"I have your results. Your PSA is minus zero-point-one, and that's very good. Your urine culture and analysis is normal, and your testosterone level is seventy-two."

I'm writing the number *seventy-two* and circling it. "What's it supposed to be?"

"Two hundred."

"Wow!"

"When you were taking your medications, it was in the twenties."

I want to ask him how long will it take to get back to normal, but I don't have the nerve, so there's only the deadness of a awkward pause.

"You're doing very nicely." He wants to reassure me.

"Thank you—I owe it all to you."

"You're welcome, Eric."

He hangs up.

And that's that. I'm numb. I should be ecstatic, but I'm anesthetized by the news. I've circled *infection, bacteria, testosterone, Diane, low seventy-two*, and the number *two hundred.*

ROUND 37

IT all started at four in the morning, and after numerous trips to the bathroom, I give up any hope of getting any sleep. Back in the day when I couldn't sleep I'd be fantasizing about the flock of nubile Catholic schoolgirls who congregate at the Oval in their tartan shirts hiked up to their navels; the NYU lovelies, long-legged, well-endowed Nordic beauties from the Midwest who live two doors down; the sexy shrink with the Angelina lips on five; or the hottie divorcée on three who has a fondness for leather halters and takes out her garbage in stilettos. In my bed, in the comfort and security of the darkness, self-love is the rhythm of the night, and eventually sleep comes as we did, Mr. Stiffy and me. But now no slapping the monkey, choking the chicken, beating the bishop, buttering the corn, or flogging the log this morning, not last night, and—if I don't do something about it—not tomorrow night.

I go into the kitchen, open up the vial of Viagra, pop a one-hundred-milliliter bluey, down it with some soy milk, and return to bed. Why did I wait five months for this? I tell myself it's because I don't have the urge—don't really care about sex; true, but I know the real reason—it won't fucking work!

Erectile dysfunction—funny, when this all started it took a backseat to death. But now let's get real—what good is getting it up if you can't *get* up? Now—that doesn't mean you shouldn't be looking at all your options with an eye to the health and well-being of the one-eyed snake. After carefully digesting the research data, tons of anecdotal evidence, but most important of all, Ira's very own and unique *happy ending,* I choose hormones, radiation, and seeds because deep, deep, deep, deep down I never doubt that Mr. Stiffy and I wouldn't be together again. What I don't count on is the precipitous drop in my testosterone (thank you Zoladexers, wherever you are) or what part Mr. Linear Accelerator 1 plays in robbing me of the will to fuck.

I know—I know both Dr. Berman and Dr. Ng strongly recommend I begin taking Viagra or Cilias right after my implants. When I confess to Dr. Ng I don't have anyone, he tells me to rent some porn or, *Just go outside and open your eyes.* I know—I know it's summertime, when the women are easy to drool over, always a wonderful wake-up time for Mr. Stiffy. Heck—all it would take is the elevator ride with just-out-of-the-shower, perfume-soaked beauties to get the snake to dance in your pants. How many times, how many times, my brothers, do I see them bending over to adjust a strap on their high heels while clutching iPods and Blackberries, mugs of steaming coffee in their free hands, sumptuous mounds of breast flesh forcing their way out of the encumbering low-cut slips that pass for sundresses? ENOUGH TIMES TO RIDE THE ELEVATOR UP AND DOWN THREE OR FOUR TIMES BEFORE I LEAVE THE BUILDING, ALL RIGHT?

Do you know what it's like to see more skin than you saw in a skin magazine when you were growing up just inches away from your face first thing in the AM—when the pecker's at his peak—and feel *bupkis*, nothing, *nada, rien?* I'll tell you what it's like—like when you've got a 105 fever and you're floating above your body, staring down at your disconnected self lying motionless on the bed and thinking—*WHAT THE FUCK?*

Come clean, Eric, tell everyone what you have in your hand now, at 10:30 a.m. It's yellow and has writing on it: *bacteria, testosterone, Diane, low seventy-two,* and the number *two hundred.* You've been staring at it the last ten days because the Floppy-Does-The-Dance-Indicator is seventy-two, up from an all-time low of twenty-something, and if push comes to shove, you think that maybe—just maybe—you can take a chance again on love—reward The Boy (as in a blast that will last)—take the Viagra. And that's why six-and-a-half hours later there's lead in the ol' pencil (okay—so it's only a nub).

ROUND 38

YOU never forget those first shots to the body, and the last thing you want is to be reminded of them, but there's another reason why I've postponed my annual checkup: I'm afraid history will repeat itself and Dr. Lombardo's going to find something else wrong with me. Like what? Well—let's start with diabetes. After all, I have gained fifteen pounds, and while I blame it on the eunuch-makers from the Planet Zoladex, it could be something worse. Then there are my swollen legs and feet. Okay—OKAY, I know I should have gone to Lombardo in June, when I first noticed it—should have shown Dr. Berman immediately, who later when I did, said it looked like water retention—agreed with me when I half-heartedly suggested I will see what Lombardo thinks—but it's a few weeks after the seeds and I'm thinking it's the steroids and when they're totally out of my system the swelling will disappear. Besides, Dr. B. doesn't seem to think it's serious. Truth—I'm just too worn out to deal with another ailment; figure I'll go native, drink coffee, eat lots of asparagus and heal myself. What I don't figure on is how, when I take off my socks at night, the indentations they make in my ankles create disturbing images of Pop's swollen feet and the meds he took to keep them from turning elephantine and exploding.

So—how come I'm here today? *"Come on, pally, lost your nerve?"* Sound familiar? It does to me. Nobody's going to call me a yellow belly every day for two months and get away with it—even if they do carry a pistolero.

The tiny office is surprisingly crowded, but I'm a little early and not planning on going anywhere, so I don't care if I've got to wait. I pull out my book, *A Fraction of the Whole.* No—it's not the title of my book or anything dealing with the loss of a body part, instead, it's one of the Booker Prize nominees (I'm reading them all), and because Dr. Lombardo and I like to turn each other on to books, I figure I'll read him the impressive first page so he can judge whether he wants to pick it up for himself. I also intend to talk up another nominee, *The White Tiger*, a brilliant first novel by a twenty-something wunderkind. Oh—I've also got a Rankin book stashed away—never enter a doctor's office without it.

I'm not particularly thrilled that neither Linda, the receptionist, nor Boy Tech greet me with enthusiasm. Am I so insecure that I need constant stroking? But everyone else seems to be getting theirs! Maybe they're regulars—really sick folks who come here all the time? *You want that?* No—but I've got cancer. Had *cancer—it's all gone—remember?* Yeah—but . . . *But—but—what?* Uhh . . . *And what's up with playing the cancer card?*

"This is new and pretty weak—even for you, pally."

I look away. Even I know when I can't face myself.

Okay, let's go over the checklist again: Take blood from the left arm, not the right; get a blood test for diabetes; show Dr. L. your swollen feet; and last, but certainly not least, make sure to tell him you just had a rectal exam.

I'm going to blame the extra weight on the hormones, maybe even on the swollen feet. (Hey, there's nothing wrong with playing the hormone card).

One last thing—give him the new PSA numbers, results of the urine tests, and tell him about the testosterone levels, but be upbeat—this is one problem you *can* blame on the boys from Planet Zoladex.

Dr. Lombardo exits his office and looks over at me. "Young man, what are you reading?"

Before I get all worked up, I remember he calls all his patients *young man* or *young woman*. I hand Dr. Lombardo the book. "Read the first page, I think you'll like it."

Right away he's nodding, laughing. "We'll talk later." He hands the book back, tells Boy Tech to get the examining room ready.

"It's all done," says Boy Tech.

"Go in Eric, I'll be in in a minute."

He returns to his office and closes the door.

Boy Tech follows me into the treatment room, instructs me to take off everything down to my socks, T-shirt, and shorts, and then he leaves. The room is cold, but I comply. I pull out my book, read a page or two (I must be relaxed, I'm actually concentrating). I hear Dr. Lombardo pull my chart off the plastic holder on the outside of the door. Showtime!

"So, young man, how have you been?"

"You know I have prostate cancer."

The words come out so effortlessly you would think I'm talking about the weather. I'm amazed at my nonchalance. Am I so blasé because I think I'm totally cured, believe cancer cells no longer live in my body—or have I accepted my condition and made peace with it?

Dr. Lombardo nods. He begins his examination. I reel off my checklist as he checks my eyes, throat, and ears and listens to my chest. When I tell him about my swollen feet he asks me to remove my socks, but finds nothing.

"Everything looks good," he says.

He wants to know what I'm doing these days, and when I tell him I'm writing a book about my cancer, mention he's in it—that I'm only saying nice things about him—he says that's good. When I tell him the title, he laughs, says that's a great choice. He describes a book he thinks I should read (*Out Stealing Horses*), asks me to come into his office after the exam is over. He leaves. Suddenly, as if lifted by a magic carpet, I rise, and hover over the table until I hear Boy Tech at the door. I gently lower myself, unfolding my legs from the lotus position as I descend until I'm sitting on the table, legs dangling off the side.

I immediately tell Boy Tech about my rolling veins and offer up my left arm so no mistakes will be made. (I saw the picture of the woman who had her hands and feet amputated by mistake.) I make small talk, remind Boy Tech of the time we met—his fourth day on the job. The boy's all business, but I do get a nod and wonder if he remembers that exam, lathering me up with electrolyte salve, placing the cold EKG electrodes on my chest, arms and legs, still thinking I was dishing him when I laughingly exclaim—*Boy, that's cold as a witch's tit!* Okay—when the lady at the CCC lathered me up during my pre-op exam, I let out an involuntary orgasmic moan, but that was different—the radiation made me do it.

I'm down with Boy Tech's misguided vibe, and when he does the EKG I'm so cool, I'm betting if you compare my EKG with George's after he took the Garcia dude to the cleaners in *Ocean's 12*, you couldn't tell the difference.

The tests are finished. I get dressed in a slow and unhurried manner and, feeling strangely calm, head for Dr. Lombardo's office. Whatever—I just have to deal with it, *tsum glik, tsum shlimazel*—for better, for worse.

Dr. Lombardo is viewing my EKG results records; he looks up when I enter and gives me a huge smile.

"Looking very good, young man."

I crack a thin one. No jumping up and clicking of heels? Maybe tomorrow— maybe tomorrow . . .

ROUND 39

I have been up since 6:00 a.m., drinking coffee, cleaning the house, and getting my Dopamine load from Dinu Lipatti. Before my cancer it's easy to close my eyes and just drift away down my electrical circuitry, which resonates in perfect harmony with each note, but for the last thirteen months a minute here or there is all I can sustain.

Today there is no time limit; each repetition is like I'm hearing it for the first time, that's how starved my circuitry is for this chemical perfection that manifests itself in the soothing rhythms of Bach's *Partita for Keyboard No. 1 in B-flat Major BMV 825*, and the other sublime pieces of Bach, Schubert, Mozart, and Scarlatti, so when Dr. Lombardo calls and gives me the good news I feel a double surge of electrical mellow yellow.

Round 40

FUNNY how you never realize you have stuff bottled up until it explodes right out of your mouth. One minute you're fine, the next you're a giant soda bottle and someone turns you upside down, shakes you, twists off the cap. *Whoosh!*

The elevator stops at six. A perky neighbor lady who always has a happy smiling face gets on and immediately gives me a big hello. She's wrapped from head to toe in a white down jacket and hood and looks like a tiny polar bear.

"Hi!"

"Hi!"

"A happy and healthy New Year to you and yours."

"You, too."

I'm pretty sure she works at a hospital. "Health is so important, isn't it?" I comment.

"Oh yes. I see that every day."

"Sloan-Kettering?"

"No—Weill Cornell—New York Presbyterian."

"I'm sorry, I forgot your name."

"Ilene."

"I'm Eric."

"Hi!"

"Hi!"

It's my plan to head to my right and over to the bank, the library, then work my way back for food and wine. She's going to her left, toward 14th Street. I need my soda bottle shook.

"Oh, I can go this way, too," I say.

"I work in the urology department. I've been there over twenty years."

She's shaking the bottle!

"I have prostate cancer." *Whoosh!* "But I'm okay."

"You look healthy."

"I feel fine. I have some side effects, but I can't really complain: hot flashes, and my testosterone level is really low.

"Have you thought about Lupron?"

Lupron—now that's really funny. I wonder how my buds from the Planet Zoladex would feel about that?

"I don't like taking drugs."

How's that for a lame excuse?

Ilene nods. "It does have some strong side effects."

We're passing residents on their way home. Heads are down, snow is flying in their faces, pasting their cheeks with white flakes. The wind is howling. Why do I think they can hear my conversation?

"I took Zoladex. It was part of my treatment. I had radiation and . . . "

"A prostatectomy . . . ?"

"No . . . Uh . . . the seeds." Why couldn't I remember more quickly?

"Seed implantation." She's nodding.

"Over at St. Vincent's. They're terrific."

"Tom in our building had it there. He told me the hospital took great care of him."

"Tom?"

"He lives with Frank. They're away a lot. He's always talking about how much he liked St. Vincent's and how they managed his side effects."

"I guess I was lucky. The radiation didn't affect me at all."

"I work for Dr. Bander. He's discovered a way to target cancer cells and kill them. No more surgery, no more radiation. Isn't that wonderful? They're doing trials on it now

"What's his name again?"

"Dr. Bander. Dr. Neil H. Bander. Look him up on the Internet."

We get to 14th Street. Ilene is going to take a cross-town bus heading west, but nothing's coming.

"I was really nervous about the biopsy. They inject Lidocaine right into the prostate to deaden the pain."

"Yep." When she says *yep*, she gives a little shake and looks like a giant bobblehead polar bear.

"The Lidocaine shot doesn't hurt, either, because they put a topical painkiller on the area."

"Yep."

"All I felt was a little pinch. Same when they take the samples from your prostate. Twelve little pinches."

"Yep, yep."

"The only thing that bothers me is they take such small samples."

"But there's lots of science behind the procedure. They pretty much know what you have, where you have it, and what stage the cancer's in. Eric, you look very healthy. God bless."

I'm feeling very religious myself. Thank God she can't see the tears for the flakes that run down my cheeks. I don't want her to leave. I want to tell her about my seed implantation, the Foley, my garbage bag—my relationship to Moses. Then there is the stuff about my bone scan, but it's too late. She's hugging me. I'm hugging her.

"Happy New Year and God bless."

"God bless."

I'm so caught up in her religious fervor that I nearly make the sign of the cross. I turn, walk toward First Avenue, and immediately find myself in the middle of five Hispanics: two adults and three teens, dressed in identical black North Face parkas. A family, happily engaged in animated conversation, all caught up in the holiday spirit. I can't help but smile. For some reason I look down at their feet. They're wearing sneakers, all of them. My mind's racing. Who the hell wears sneakers in the snow?

I'm no longer an upside-down soda bottle.

ROUND 41

SOMETHING is moving in my right eye. I first notice it yesterday, while I'm typing away on the computer, and I think it's a fly, so I try to swat it. It's so small, this thing that zooms by, that I figure it's on the monitor—some kind of pixilation? Maybe that's why I let the incident pass. Now that I think of it, this silly thing may have occurred before— days, weeks ago, I can't be sure; the events are unclear and float out of range, just like the thing in my eye, and when I reach for the memory, consciousness and unconsciousness repel one another, as when two positively charged objects come in contact.

Today, it's more distracting, especially in the bright light of my bathroom, where this thing is bigger, darker, and faster than a speeding bullet. *Hey, I thought I'm Iron Man—I don't need no Superman references.*

Maybe I'm tired? Maybe it's a little more serious, say, a symptom of a cataract? There's laser surgery for that, and nowadays it's no big thing. I even think it's painless. Well, maybe not—probably have to have a local. I'm seeing needles into my eye. This isn't good.

My dad had it done. Actually, I think he may have had both eyes done. I'm not sure how old he was—his seventies maybe, maybe not; maybe he was my age when he had the procedure. I don't remember ever seeing him with his eyes bandaged. I would have seen it if he was here in New York; maybe he was living in Atlantic City or down in Florida? He probably was with Miss L. She called me when he had his pacemaker put in, why wouldn't she call when he had laser surgery?

Next up the scale of terrible things is a detached retina. I don't think I have that. I know that's extremely painful and I have no pain. Perhaps this is only a partial tear? I'll have to go on the Internet, check it out. I'll wait until tomorrow. In the meantime, I take two Aleve; they will relax me now and help me to get a good night's sleep.

There's something else nagging at me—cancer, brain tumor. I had a sharp pain in my head last week. I thought it was from the cold, sinus headache, but now . . . Cancer—it got out of the prostate and it's in my brain. How could that be? The bone and PET scans are clean. Cancer can't grow that fast—can it? Right? Right!

The Aleve is relaxing me to the point that I'm able to read for only thirty minutes before my eyes finally are so heavy, I put the book down, close the light, and go to sleep. But I have to pee first.

I postpone my Sunday ritual of going out for coffee and a muffin and go to the Internet. I look up cataracts and the symptoms don't match. THANK YOU, GOD! Pain, double or blurred vision, some nasty stuff here. I get the shivers and quickly get back onto Google. I'm not going to type in "floaters" because that reminds me of what they call the bodies they find in the river. More shivers. I think a minute. I type in "black spots in the eye" (not very original, but accurate), and low and behold as I'm typing "black spots in . . ." *black spots in vision, skin, face, roses,* and *black spots in the eyes* appear; praise be!

I click on *black spots in the eyes* and I am rewarded with an entire page of diagnoses. I quickly scan the descriptions.

"I see black spots! Please, help me! Do I have some disease? These black spots appear all of sudden and disappear without any reason."

"Black spots or 'spider webs' that seem to float in the vision in a cluster or alone; spots that move or remain suspended in one place."

The latter is posted by Stlukeseye.com (the hospital?) and also seems less frantic (don't worry, I'll check the former link—birds of a feather, etc.). The page comes up immediately. I read until I get to *"This is called posterior vitreous detachment (PVD), a very common, usually harmless condition."*

I'm so relieved, I forget about going out and decide to make myself a cup of coffee. I can kick myself for not going to the Web sooner and sparing myself an evening of anxiety.

ROUND 42

WITHOUT a doubt, I made the right choice in coming to see Dr. P., who reminds me of H. B. Warner, the wise immortal of *Lost Horizon*. His private office is a cross between Holmes's front room at 221B Baker Street and Louis Pasteur's lab, and will most likely be donated to the Smithsonian after the doc lifts his final eyelid. I'm immediately feeling at home.

"Take a seat." He checks out my information sheet.

I check out the massive bookshelves. "Are those titles in Latin?"

"You're a writer. What have you written?"

I wish I could translate *The Yummy Hunter's Guide* into the language of Francis of Assisi. "Uhh—a health book, but now I'm writing one about my battle with prostate cancer."

He nods. "I had it, too . . ." He looks at me, smiles, and I get the oddest feeling he can see my future—and it's all good.

It's been awhile since I've had an ophthalmologist check out my eyes (I usually go to a local eyeglass store), but even so, I don't ever remember anyone being so thorough. The upshot: some floaters in my right eye and a cataract in my left; not to worry about either, unless the cataract hinders my ability to see.

"Come back in two weeks; I'd like to check out these results, and perhaps write you out a new eyeglass prescription."

I'm on the street walking quickly so I won't be late to Dr. Berman (three-month checkup), my eyes blurry and teary. I'm unable to read the time off my watch, or see it on the face of my cell phone. I have a feeling I'm not going to make it in time. Not to worry, I told Dr. B's receptionist I might be late.

Out on Park Ave., people are walking around in shirtsleeves. I know the recession hit the rich hard, but I didn't expect them to be selling the clothes off their backs. As I cross the street, I hear the voice of a WINS radio announcer coming loud and clear from an open car window. It's fifty-three degrees. So it's not the recession. The station at 77th and Lex is crowded with local high-school kids going home, but I walk to the extreme south end of the platform and the crowd thins. I'm lucky; A downtown 6 train arrives within minutes. I rush into the first car and grab a seat. At the next stop a fresh horde push their way in. A young Moslem woman, completely encased in a black, stands above me.

"Would you like to sit?"

She nods. She keeps her head down, avoids eye contact as I stand over her.

I get off at 42nd and immediately catch the express on the other side of the platform.

I'm at Dr. B's in record time—not that I can easily read the clock in the reception area to confirm this, with blurry eyes and eyelids that weight a ton. The waiting area is empty. Is it the economy? Could men be so psyched out by the downward spiral that they're disregarding the aching pee-pee, hitting the bars, or just hitting Mr. Floppy against the wall? Ouch!

I sign in, make my excuses for being ten minutes late, but the receptionist tells me it doesn't matter. She looks over to the examining rooms.

"He doesn't have anyone waiting."

I sit. Five minutes later a young Latina tech leads me into an examining room.

"Hello."

"Hello."

I recognize her. She's sweet and good with the needle. I was hoping to get Lovely Blonde Nightingale, but I'm sure she's hiding from me.

The tech notices my eyes.

"I've just come from an eye exam."

"I can tell. Your pupils are huge."

"I took the train down here. I hope nobody thought I was weird—on drugs?"

She's smiling, shaking her head. "Pupils normally enlarge in a dark area, for instance, when you go into a room without lights."

"It wasn't that dark—it was a subway car, a packed subway car; was that the reason the Moslem lady didn't look up at me? Why didn't I wear shades?

The tech surprises me when she puts the BP cuff over my sleeve. We both watch the screen. It's blurry, but I think I can make out the numbers: 136/84.

"That's good," she says, repeating those exact numbers.

She unwrapping the cuff, putting it away, her back is now to me.

"The last time I think it was one-twenty over eighty." I'm nervous and hope my voice doesn't give me away.

She half-turns, smiles sweetly, showing me a nice set of perfectly matched white uppers and lowers. "Are you nervous?"

"No."

"Did you run over here?"

"I picked up the pace, but I didn't run."

"That's the reason, then."

She smiles. I can't.

"What do you weigh?"

"One-hundred-seventy-five." That's comes out quickly and without self-censorship. I'm surprised I'm no longer lying about this personal obscenity. I'm ashamed of myself for my lack of portion control, and more importantly, the laziness that prevents me from exercising is behavior I bitterly despise. I'm always using the hormones as an excuse, but there's a limit to how long you can lie to yourself—at least I hope there is.

"I have to take your blood."

"Okay—but you have to use the left arm. I have rolling veins."

I'm so enamored with my ability to remember this I can't help but giggle. The tech smiles back, but I know in my heart of hearts she thinks I'm strange.

The bloodletting is painless, and in less than five minutes Dr. Berman enters. We exchange pleasantries.

"Are you still on the Flomax?"

"Nope. I stopped that way back in September."

"That's good. How about erections?"

"All's quiet on the Southern Front."

"Are you taking anything for it?"

"A few times I took Cilias, one time a Viagra, but nothing." I may be exaggerating on the Cilias, but I'm grasping for straws here. "I am getting more feeling in my penis. I'm stimulating myself." I can't believe I'm saying this, but I'm proud the desire is back and I want to boast about my heightened sexuality, limited that it is. "I'm also dreaming about sex."

"Are you waking up with an erection?"

"No."

"Would you like a suppository?"

I'm thinking, *Up my you-know-what?*

As if he's reading my mind, he says "You insert it into the penis."

Confusion changes to horror. I can feel Mr. Floppy folding up into my abdomen.

"I'll pass."

"Have you tried Levitra?"

"No." I shake my head for emphasis.

"I'll give you some."

"Thank you."

He examines my abdomen, then I follow his instructions and turn to my left—it's muscle tightening time. There are a few *oohs*, *ahhs*, and winces, and it seems to go on forever, but you don't have to cry for me, Argentina.

"It's still swollen, isn't it?" I ask.

"It'll take a full year for it to come down. You said you're off the Flomax?"

"Yes—since last September."

"What is your frequency?"

AM or FM? My neurons are giggling. Oh, how easy it is to return to flippancy when you're not afraid of dying. "Seems normal during the day. At night it varies—sometimes every two hours, sometimes three, four-hour intervals. I think it depends on how much liquid I take in and when. The later I drink, the more frequently I pee."

He's nodding, writing as I speak. I'm really concentrating. I don't want to forget anything.

"Should I take a urine test?"

"Yes. When was the last time you urinated?"

"Three hours ago."

"I also want to check your flow."

"In that machine—in the bathroom at the end of the hall?"

"Yes." He closes the thick manila folder and hands me a small box of tissues. "I'll see you in my office." He leaves. Nobody likes to see a grown man wipe.

I use up half the tissues, leave one in to prevent the residue of jelly he inserts for his smooth ride in from leaking all over my shorts—a half-assed measure (no pun intended), but like they say, an ounce of prevention . . . I'm always nervous I'm going to see blood afterwards, however, I'm figuring the odds are low since I didn't see anything, even after my operation. I wonder if I should look. I think. I smile. I relax. I look. *Bupkis*, nothing, *nada, rien*! I am Iron Man!

I scan the room. I think I see the peak of a fedora, but it's nothing—maybe a floater.

Out in the hall I spot Lovely Blonde Nightingale sitting in a tiny room full of lab equipment. I suddenly forget where the bathroom is located.

"Where do I go to measure my flow?"

She smiles, points to the bathroom located directly in front of me.

"Okay, I knew that."

We both laugh. I wonder if she's seen Marlowe?

I enter the bathroom. The pee machine is right next to the sink. It's a large white plastic funnel hooked up to a meter, and a thin pipe I assume leads to the building's plumbing. I remember the last time it took awhile to pee and the stream was decent, but not anything to write home about, although I was pleased it wasn't old-fogey weak. Now I'm confident I'm going to unleash a mighty jet that will rock the meter to its core.

Why can't I go? *Relax, will you?* This is surprising. *A few deep breaths, but not too deep, there's the smell of urine in the air, remember?* I stare down into the cavernous mouth of the uroflowmetry. Can't expect to go on command when someone's just played with your prostate and everything down there is all jazzed up; give it another couple a seconds before you freak. There it goes. Nice and strong and steady, maybe not the jet stream I'm hoping for, but good enough.

Soon I'm in Dr. Berman's office, and he's writing more stuff in my file. In front of him is an electronic readout of my flow.

"Your stream is very good, much better than the last time you were here." He hands me a box of Levitra and a capsule marked Viagra. I stuff it into my pocket. "I'll see you in three months."

I reach out and shake his hand. "Thank you doctor, thank you very much."

"You're welcome, Eric."

I turn, stare for an instant at all his awards and the many pictures of his family. Once more, I'm relieved—rejuvenated, almost. I've again dodged the bullet and it's an incredible-lightness-of-being moment. I want to thank Dr. B. in a more effusive manner, but at moments like these I can never find the words.

I go to the reception desk and tell her he wants to see me in three months. She scans her calendar, mentions a date. I nod. She writes it out on his card and hands it over.

I forgot something. I turn and step into his office. He's on the phone and looks up.

"You'll test my testosterone level, right?"

"I wasn't going to, but I will."

"Do you need more blood?"

"No, you're fine."

"Okay, see ya."

He nods, goes back to his phone. I'm suddenly feeling guilty about being so rude. But he *did* look up. He *did* acknowledge me.

Will you just get the heck out of here? I turn, follow the way of my neurons, and feel I'm on the verge of a Bruce Willis moment of triumph.

ROUND 43

THE phone rings, and I see by the caller ID it's Dr. Berman. It flashes through my brain that he's calling a day early.

"Shit, shit, and double-shit!"

"Hello, it's Dr. Berman, and I have your results. Your PSA is again very good, minus point zero one, and your testosterone is one-oh-one; that's up from seventy-two, so things are progressing well."

I'm momentarily stunned. "Ah . . . the PSA, it's the same as last time?"

"Yes. You're doing very well. I'll see you in three months."

Another thank-you will not cut it. My instincts are to kiss the god's feet, or at the very least do a couple hundred genuflections, but over the phone that's pretty hard.

"You're the best, Doctor, the very best. Thank you."

It's a poor imitation of Tina's jubilant rendition, but remember I'm on the phone; that doesn't mean once I hang up I don't start dancing around my living room like a fool.

"You're simply the best, better than all the rest, better than anyone, anyone I've ever met!"

Round 44

Tuesday, February 10, 2009, 2:45 p.m. *Last one standing . . .*

FUNNY how time flies when you're not having your walnut messaged, punched full of holes, radiated, or seeded. I leave myself an hour for my cross-town journey, but I know from experience that when I start taking my street photos I can foul up my timetable, and today's no different. So when I get to Sixth Avenue and check my watch, I realize I have to pick up the pace if I'm to get to my appointment on time.

As I get closer to St. Vinny's, I study each pedestrian, looking for signs that they, too, are fellow patients. Women and men with wigs and toupees are obvious choices, but guys like me are more difficult to spot. In this neighborhood, sad, downtrodden expressions are a dead giveaway, although the city's faltering economy could be the cause. More often it's the pasty white skin; dark circles under the red-rimmed, puffy eyes; or the drawn, gaunt look; although hollow cheeks can be a sign of AIDS rather than prostate cancer—however, I imagine the late stages of my or any other cancer would similarly ravage the body.

I smile at everybody. It's a compassionate smile. It's one that says, *I have it, too, and I know what you're going through.* At least this is the message I want my brain to send to my facial muscles. I have no idea if it's an accurate translation, but when I get an identical smile, I imagine two ships passing in the night, crews flashing messages back and forth, each recognizing their lonely plight, each finding solace in their kinship.

I breeze past the front desk.

"Good afternoon, gentlemen." The two male gatekeepers look up. I throw them a salute. "I'm going to see Dr. Ng."

They smile. I'm bouncing with joy as I enter the waiting room. On my left, sitting on one of the extremely narrow leather benches, is a very sad-looking woman in her mid-forties. Behind her is the Breast Cancer Center. The last thing I want to do is disrespect her emotional state. I dial down the smile and nod. To my right, on an identical leather bench, is an elderly couple, I'm guessing from an Eastern European country. They stare at my professional-looking Nikon D90 dangling from my right hand (*no more point-and-shoot for me, boyo*). I nod, smile, and quickly make a left and head down the familiar white corridor.

Connie's sitting at the first desk and Elizabeth is sitting at the second station. I point to Connie and do my favorite *you, you, you* De Niro imitation from *Analyze This*. We share hugs and hellos.

"I'm here to see Dr. Ng for my six-month checkup. I know, I know registration—right? Registration—right!"

I'm back in ten, hand Connie the necessary paperwork, and I ask if she and Elizabeth would mind if I took their photos. They happily agree. I snap off a few individual shots, then ask them to pose together for one. I show them the results on the LED screen; they like them, want more, but first have to primp, check their looks in their hand mirrors. I take a few more and everyone is happy.

While I wait for my appointment, I make myself some fancy flavored coffee from the fancy coffee machine (although it takes me a few seconds to remember how to use it). I grab a fruit bar and take a seat. I'm never here at this time, still I'm surprised the place isn't jam-packed like in the morning. As usual, there are numerous Chinese: two elderly couples and three middle-aged men. Next to me is a well-dressed, Hispanic man in his late thirties or early forties, softly cursing under his breath. It's obvious he's been waiting a while and is growing more impatient by the minute, showing his frustration when Connie or one of the nurses calls another patient to go in for their treatment. This is the first time I've seen anyone here show dissatisfaction or impatience, except when one of the machines goes down and appointments back up and a few patients grumble about being late for work while others simply postpone treatments.

I finish my coffee, go in to pee, a little anxious my name will be called, and even though I don't hear anyone ask for me, the moment I leave the bathroom I run into a nurse who tells me she hopes I'm not trying to avoid her because she knows all about me and was in the operating room for my implants. *Oh—so you're the sadist I have to thank for going home with a catheter up my you-know-what?* I say nothing.

I follow her to the treatment area and see Dr. Ng along the way. I saw him for a brief moment when I first came into the reception area, and immediately noticed something different. He's got hair! He slips away before I can say anything, but now, as I walk by, I point to my own mop.

"Cool."

He smiles.

The nurse wants to weigh me, and it comes out to one-eighty-two.

"Should I take my shoes off—I can take my shoes off?" Sweat covers my forehead.

The nurse senses my fragile grip on reality. "Let's make it one-seventy-eight."

My lens goes from 120mm to a 18mm wide angle, but it's not enough to capture the entire room in one shot, so I take a few from different angles and get the desired results. I don't remember the paintings of clouds and I don't see the diagram of the prostate. Is it possible I've never been in this is treatment room?

The nurse leaves the door open. I can see Dr. Ng walking back and forth in the hallway, quietly conversing with the nursing staff. I can hear the nurse that weighed me, weighing someone else. One-seventy-five. It's the Impatient Man. She ushers him into the room next to me, and asks him whether he wants her to keep the door open or closed.

"You better keep it open."

His tone leads me to believe that if she doesn't comply he'll pull out an AK-47 and starts shooting. I can just see the clever *NY Post* headline: "Man Riddled with Cancer Riddles Cancer Center." I didn't see any weapons when he was sitting next to me, but he could be concealing them in his waistband; a couple of fully automatic twelve-clip handguns could do serious damage. *What am I thinking? Don't you have anything better to think about?* Well, it can happen. He does look really pissed off. *Yeah . . . but . . .*

Dr. Ng enters. He's smiling broadly. I rise and shake his hand. I'm saved from another one of my crazy migraines. He pores over my file as I give him a blow by blow. He's dismayed I just saw Dr. Berman.

"It makes no sense to give you two exams so close to each other, unless you enjoy them."

"Only if you take me dancing and buy me a nice meal afterwards—oh, and flowers would be nice."

He does a double take and we both laugh.

"We can take this show on the road and call ourselves The Smart Asses." I want to add, *And we'll wipe up*, but I smartly censor myself—cancer can do that to you.

We spend about fifteen minutes shooting the breeze. He fills me in on hospital gossip. I tell him how I'm recommending him and Dr. Berman to anyone who's got prostate problems. We talk some more about my general health, mention that thing on my nose, that it's a mild form of skin cancer and not related to my prostate and how it's no big thing (now that I know what it is, IT'S NO FUCKING BIG THING), that it's going to be removed by a MOHS surgeon.

"Happens all the time. Stay out of the sun."

"Yeah, I know."

There's a pause as he continues to write in my file, so I nonchalantly bring up Mr. Stiffy and tell him I'm starting to get that loving feeling again. I could be more precise, refer to these new sensations as muscle sensitivity, erectile excitement, a little bit of hardness (that's too extreme)—a Mr. Stiffy awakening? I'm going to leave out the humiliating desire to self-serve (been there, done that with Dr. Berman).

"You're having sex. That's great."

"Well, not exactly."

"You're taking the Viagra and watching porn?"

"Well, not exactly."

Dr. Ng reads me like the top line of an eye chart.

"My testosterone level's up from fifty-something to one-oh-one!"

"You need to get those nerves and muscles working."

I smile. Berman hasn't told him I'm into playing the old skin flute again.

We go on to talk about his new hairstyle and living his downtown life. The simple act of talking with my oncologist about everyday stuff puts me on such a high, that when I leave I know my body's experienced a healing as curative as if he had given me a new miracle drug. I wonder if in a past life Dr. Ng was a shaman? I can imagine him putting his healing hands on me, hear him reciting a litany of restorative incantations in a mystical language, while I lie naked on a straw mat, a blazing fire illuminating the magical scene. Oh yeah, there's ominous rhythmic chanting, accompanied by beating drums—have to have drums beating.

I'm two blocks east of the hospital when I come out of my daydream. I'm walking briskly, and other than the extra weight and a bit of stiffness in my joints, my body feels pretty good. Lugging around the extra weight can be attributed to eating like a pig, stiffness from a lack of exercise, or maybe a little arthritis; nothing really abnormal or scary going on. It's as if my body has no memory of the cancer and is signaling ditto to my brain, causing my neurotransmitters to convey normal happy thoughts and smiley-boy faces.

Unfortunately, this lovely scenario is marred when I look around the neighborhood and remember the time I didn't know if I could hold my water for another second. I know the radiation has left my body, but did it ever radiate out into these sidewalks, store fronts, commercial and residential buildings, even zap the vast amounts of dog poop I have to deftly sidestep—not only the poop in this radiated nabe, but all poop, everywhere and anywhere I walked in the Big Apple?

The crowd noise in Union Square blots out this crazy brain chatter before a pile-of-poop-in-the-bedroom-without-a-scooper migraine brings me to my knees. I'm forced to pay strict attention or else get trampled by the whirl of people on a mission to find the most delicious head of organic romaine, Bibb, or Celtuce (look it up, I had to). It's the farmers' market! They come from all over, looking for the freshest of fresh, squeezing, fondling. The most frightening are the over-seventy group, using bicycles fitted with enormous baskets as battering rams to get from one stall to another.

I tip my hat to Marlowe, who is now standing over a huge display of roasted and salted nuts. He cracks a smile as he cracks a walnut in his huge mitt.

"Yippee-ki-yay, motherfucker!"